Also by Jake Steinfeld

Power Living by Jake
Don't Quit!

STRONG!

GET

Body by Jake's Guide to
Building Confidence,
Muscles, and a Great
Future for Teenage Guys

Jake Steinfeld

A Fireside Book
Published by Simon & Schuster
New York London Toronto Sydney Singapore

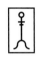

FIRESIDE
Rockefeller Center
1230 Avenue of the Americas
New York, NY 10020

FIRESIDE and colophon are registered trademarks
of Simon & Schuster, Inc.

For information about special discounts for bulk purchases,
please contact Simon & Schuster Special Sales:
1-800-456-6798 or business@simonandschuster.com

Designed by Lisa Stokes

Manufactured in the United States of America

1   3   5   7   9   10   8   6   4   2

Library of Congress Cataloging-in-Publication Data is available.

ISBN 0-7432-2477-9

This publication contains the opinions and ideas of its author. It is intended to provide helpful and informative material on the subjects addressed in the publication. It is sold with the understanding that the author and publisher are not engaged in rendering medical, health, or any other
kind of personal professional services in the book. The reader should consult his or her medical,
health, or other competent professional before adopting any of the suggestions in this book or
drawing inferences from it.

The author and publisher specifically disclaim all responsibility for any liability, loss or risk,
personal or otherwise, which is incurred as a consequence, directly or indirectly, of the use and
application of any of the contents of this book.

ACKNOWLEDGMENTS

Some Special People, Some Special Thoughts

Jan "Jan-ola" Miller—Let's just say, "No Jan, no book!!" The Superagent.

Phil "Philly" Scotti—He will not quit until Body by Jake is a household brand name, worldwide!

David "Zelly" Zelon—From Zolty to Zabo to Yokomo to Bobbo, twenty-five years of training together. Check out the factor!

Dr. Bob "The Animal" Goldman—The smartest guy I know, from a brain-resuscitation machine to record-setting handstand push-ups!

Jay "Jaydo" Silverman—They don't make better guys, or better photographers. (Cover shot: Central Park, 104 degrees, 100 percent humidity. Jaydo: cool as a cucumber.)

Bob "Bob-O" Lieberman—The man who has taken care of my business since 1980.

ACKNOWLEDGMENTS

vi

Ethan "E" Boldt—A great writer, with great courage and a Don't Quit! attitude. (He also loves flying in private planes.)

Dominick "D-Man" Anfuso—Thanks for your unwavering support and belief in my vision.

Joy "My Mom" Steinfeld—The woman who taught me that the world is a good place and, yes, that the good guys will always win!

To my wife, Tracey, and my kids, Morgan,
Nick, Zach, and Luke—you make me so proud to be a
husband and a dad! I love you guys forever!!

CONTENTS

CONTENTS

GETSTRONG!

INTRODUCTION:
DREAMS WORK

Maybe you're like I was: You go to bed every night dreaming about having big muscles, playing guitar on stage in front of thousands, getting the girl, dunking in a big game, gaining admittance to a top university; and then you wake up. There are no muscles, no concert arena, no dunking, and no acceptance letters. Oh, and no girl, either.

Let me help you to change that and make those dreams a reality. In this book, I will show you that if you will give your dreams *power* by inviting them into your day, then your dreams will come true.

It might sound funny, but one day in high school, I had a really vivid daydream: I saw myself doing biceps curls in front of fifty thousand screaming fans at Madison Square Garden. I decided, then and there, to put that vision into action, and I've never been the same since. Suddenly, by lifting a weight, I also lifted myself out of the rut I'd been in. All my dreams that had never seen the light of day—looking lean, dating a girl named Barbara, and being my high school's basketball star—now had a fighting chance.

It took me a while to achieve those dreams, however. You see, I wasn't just another nervous fourteen-year-old freshman. It was worse. I was a fat kid with a stutter. My best friend was Pizza Pie, but I couldn't even get on the phone to order one up! I was overweight and out of shape, and I had a nasty stutter to boot.

What changed this? The fact that I dared to dream, then dared to chase those dreams. I knew that my body and brain were capable of not only better things, but of greatness—in all the different parts of my life. I knew that I needed to train hard to get there . . . to muscles, to confidence, to my future.

In fact, I worked so hard at my dreams that I became the first trainer in Hollywood, a TV personality, and a successful businessman. One guy I trained had his dreams work pretty well, too. He launched a movie studio called DreamWorks. He's my pal Steven Spielberg, whom I call Wiels.

If you decide to get with me now, then you, too, will accomplish as many feats as you are willing to dream. First, we'll start with your body, which my training advice will make strong and muscular. Meanwhile, your mind will set out on the most powerful trip imaginable—a trip that will never end.

▪ The Rapadoo ▪

The Rap-a-what? That's the lingo of my youth in Baldwin, New York. You already know I'm not a teenager, so I won't try words like "jiggy" and "whas-sup" on for size. Okay, even those words are out! See why I'm not going to try?

You will hear the same rapadoo—motivational speak—that I have given to all my clients. I showed these people how to exercise their bodies and minds in new ways. No longer were they working out only to better their physiques, but my encouragement enabled them to take on other challenges in their lives, including in their careers and in their relationships. Many of them catapulted to greatness or are on their way. When you listen to me and my rapadoo, you will be, too.

My rapadoo really took off in Los Angeles in my early twenties, when I helped a few people, most of whom were in the entertainment industry in Hollywood and some of whom were household names, to get into great shape. To my surprise, I was able to get them into almost as good shape as me (you heard me right—I always had to be more fit than my clients, no matter how competitive they were)! I had found my calling. I founded my own fitness motivation business, which spawned the entire industry of personal fitness training.

Before long, top directors, producers, and actors were knocking my door down trying to get me as their trainer. They all wanted the same thing: to reach goals they couldn't reach on their own. Now, with this book in your hand, you've got me as your trainer. What do *you* want to work on? . . . Let's go!

▪ In Your Shoes ▪

You might look at where I am now and think that we have nothing in common. After all, I've been fortunate to be involved in many endeavors, from creating the personal training industry to books and videos and infomercials to launching TV networks to founding a sports league, and you are a guy who is just launching himself into adult life.

If you think that, then just consider who I was at age fourteen: the chubby kid who cou-cou-could-dn't get a word out. Yep, I've been there—even if you haven't. I know the teenage years can be brutal.

I'm not one of those guys who says, "Just wait until you clear your teens, life gets so much better," or "I was miserable as a teenager, but look at me now!" Instead, I want you to know that I changed my life *as* a teenager, not years later.

It began one day down in my basement, where I was doing my social studies homework. Well, actually, I was just highlighting my homework, because I didn't know how to study. I was looking around the room, listening to the radio, thinking of ways not to study, when out of the corner of my eye, I spied some old weights on the laundry room shelf.

Next, I got off my fat buttissimo and got those weights down. I slapped them onto the barbell, and boom! Finally, something that made sense! I put on some tunes to get my blood pumping and tossed up some curls. While I exercised, I envisioned those fifty thousand fans at Madison Square Garden I told you about. I heard them screaming for me to do another rep, then another. When I finished, I was in a better mood than I'd been in for a long time. I certainly burned more calories than I had in ages!

Until then, not only did I know that I didn't fit in at school, but I also knew that I didn't *fit* into me! I didn't get who I was. It wasn't until I figured that out that I went places. My muscles began to grow, along with my confidence. Because you have this book, you can look forward to increased strength and confidence—and it will happen because *you* will make it happen!

The first thing you want probably isn't the moon, but something much more simple: to feel great. When you put on your clothes, you want to feel muscular, in control, and full of hope. You can do that in two ways: through a lot of bench presses, certainly, but also from putting into practice all the lessons in this book. That's how you will become strong physically *and* mentally.

▪ Putting You to the Test ▪

Don't worry, you're not going to fill in any ovals on a bubble sheet or do the shuttle run in your P.E. class. My tests are ones that you will take completely by yourself and will bring out the best in you—if not now, then certainly later.

The first test will be very simple and requires you only to stand in front of a mirror. I'll ask you how you see yourself, first physically and then mentally. Maybe you're more sticklike than bricklike, or you have more ripples of fat than muscle. Perhaps you are very shy or have a quick temper. It takes real honesty to admit where you need help, but when you answer my questions bravely, you will be on your way to taking care of those problems.

The next test is called MQ, or Muscle Quotient. Just as the IQ test measures your intelligence, the MQ tests measure your muscles. I devised MQ so you can see exactly what your muscles are capable of at this moment—speed, power, strength, endurance, flexibility, and so on—with eight tests. After finding out your score, you can plug it into a chart to see how you fare against your peers. Now you have a starting point. Where will you and your score go? You'll be so pumped to find out, you'll actually want to take this test—unlike any other—again and again!

Maybe you don't have the genetics of Shaq or the kind of business mind belonging to Bill Gates, but you have many talents—that nobody else has. I'm here to bring them out and make them work for you. I wasn't a super athlete or boy genius, but gradually I noticed that I had other unique talents that might work pretty well for me. Once I began using those talents, my belief in myself grew even more.

The potential is there, inside of you—to boost your MQ, ace your tests, get your dream girl, go to the college you want. I want you first to believe in that potential and then go all out to tap it. Success doesn't happen by chance; it happens because you're making it happen.

▪ Your Route to Muscle and More ▪

There will be no more watching from the sidelines; you're going to get in the game with my Get Strong! workout. It's where your journey to your great future starts. One hour long, it will challenge you more than any other fitness experience you've ever had. Designed especially for you, this groundbreaking workout targets your muscles in a different way each week, in order to maximize your muscle power and size. As a result, you'll get more out of it than you thought possible—sure, you'll toughen up your body, but you'll also toughen up your mind.

Are you thinking, "Jake, that's great, but I don't even have a clue how to work out, let alone how to do a biceps curl"? Then you've got the right book in your hands. I'll lead you every step of the way, and I won't start you out too hard. If, instead, your thought is, "Chief, I've lifted for years, so this is going to be too easy," hey, buddy, I had you in mind just as much. You've never trained like this, believe me, and I will show you how to ratchet it up after you get the hang of it.

Building your muscles and confidence isn't simply a matter of getting fit, however; you also need some important people on your side, whom I call the Go-To People. Even if it's just one person, a Go-To plays a huge role in your life—someone whom you can always depend on; who understands your goals and helps you achieve them; who doesn't mind giving you a firm shove in the back when it's called for!

Another helper in your desire for better muscle is food. Chances are that what you take in right now doesn't do much to boost your training efforts and results. In Chapter 9, you will learn the keys to eating for muscle, energy, and enjoyment—including how to eat exactly for your body type.

Rather than sapping your energies, training helps you do more, with more passion, each day. Once you start training with me regularly, you will see great changes inside and outside yourself. I'll ask you to invite your goals into the workout, so that much more than your body benefits. As your muscles broaden, so will your horizons. You'll see!

GET STRONG WITH THESE SIDEBARS!

Housed in sidebars throughout the book are secrets and stories that I've picked up over the years. They provide you with additional tips, tales, habits, and warnings that will greatly aid you in achieving your goals.

· Stumbling . . . to Success: inspiring real-life stories about how famous friends and I went through some rough patches before hitting success.

· Power Habit: you can never have enough good habits, and these are the cream of the crop. Learn how to put them in your arsenal.

· Dream Extreme: there's only one way to dream, and that's big. I will share some great tales of shooting for the stars—and getting there.

· Muscle Maker: my workout will do tons for your muscles, while these sidebars will inspire you further with stories and methods about how to push it even more.

· Reality Check: normally, you hear this phrase used negatively, as if to say, "Reality limits you." Well, I'm going to tell you some stories about how reality can be phenomenal!

· Training Trip-Up: there are some training practices that will only get in the way of your progress. I'll show you what to watch out for.

· Don't Quit Poem: the poem that inspired me when I was fourteen and still invigorates me today.

▪ Leading and Speeding to Your Goals ▪

If you spend most of your day following others around, you most likely won't find your goal anytime soon. Instead of being a passenger, I urge you to seize the reins as you gallop to your goals. Becoming a leader in the classroom, on a sports team, and at home paves the way. To do that effectively, you'll need to clear some hurdles along the way.

In my view, there's no goal worth having if it doesn't require hard work and resilience. Obstacles can make your life hell, or you can treat them as opportunities to make yourself stronger and smarter. The only way to do that is to face them head on. Fear should be faced the same way. A natural emotion, fear can either cripple you at the knees or energize you to steamroll it and achieve more than you would have if it hadn't existed at all! We'll examine techniques for ensuring that the latter will be the result, not the former.

Maybe you've suffered some serious setbacks in the past. Maybe a huge obstacle looms in your path right now. Neither will faze you when you get with me and believe that you have what it takes to overcome those challenges. Problems and people can test your mettle, your character, your body, and your brain. I can't wait to show you how to meet those challenges!

In school, you learn from your teachers and coaches about how to be a success in anything from French class to football—and what exercises and homework are necessary for you to be tops in your class or on your team. However, one simple lesson is often skipped over: Success is a decision that you make.

When I use that word "success," I'm not referring to P. Diddy–like wealth and celebrity—unless that's what you're gunning for. Success means achieving *whatever* you set out to achieve, whether it's in sports or social work. It's crucial to know what that goal is, because setting goals gives you the direction and drive you need to arrive at success in the first place. You'll feel more determined, because you'll not only know what you're going after, but you will also be aware of every step you'll have to climb before you can get to that goal. Meanwhile, the fears, failures, and rejections will seem like minor nuisances.

I'm giving you the tools for success, and you will supply the effort and the commitment. As you gain experience using these tools—the workout, the "power habits," the leadership skills—you will also gain confidence in what you do and where you go. Your rate of success will increase, along with your future prospects. You will be ready for every curveball that life throws you.

▪ One Last Question Before You Start ▪

My message isn't about getting twenty-inch biceps (but don't count that out!). It's about feeling better about yourself and taking control of your life—first physically, then mentally. It worked for me, and it will work for you.

Before we can begin, I have one question: Will you commit? When you do, then there will be no limits to who you'll become and what you'll accomplish. I'm serving up the juice, but if you don't drink it, it's worth nothing. Chapter 1 is your first glass. Drink it up! Don't quit!

Every client I've ever trained—from big-name directors and actors to lesser-known ones—was ready to work hard to achieve a great body, even if the body itself wasn't convinced yet. That's why they hired me. Many of them weren't prepared for their minds to strain as much as their muscles did—strain, then expand! By the end of our first training session together, not only had their muscles been through their best workout ever, so had their minds.

Chapter 1 is your first training session, and you won't even touch a weight. You will experience the same exhilarating mental sensations that my clients did and, like them, come back for more! I'm not going to be the drill sergeant type who berates you and gets in your ear on every opportunity, even if I could jump out of this book and train alongside you. Instead, I'll be the guy to push you when the time is right and pull back the reins when it's not. My aim is to pump you up—physically and mentally—not to put you down.

First, I want you to spill your guts—your dreams and fears, successes and failures—before you spill them on the training floor. You probably have many questions about how to better your body, your mind, and your future; I have the answers.

So, are you ready to listen? Are you ready for the rapadoo? Before I ever shared this motivational lingo with my clients and now with you, I used it on myself. At fourteen, I was fat, I stuttered, and—though it's hard to imagine!—my confidence was on a permanent vacation.

Life as a teenager is tough enough without looking and sounding as I did. However, by the end of that year, and especially by the end of high school, I looked and sounded like the guy I had always wanted to be. At the same time, I set myself in motion toward bigger goals.

How'd I do it? The same way you're going to do it: Look no further than inside your own head. Look to your dreams.

▪ Put Your Dreams to Work ▪

To many, a "dreamer" is a guy lost in the clouds, and to be called one is almost an insult. To me, however, it's a great compliment! I've proudly worn that tag since I was young, just as I've always imagined bigger and greater things than what surrounded me.

Whenever I mowed my parents' lawn—a job I was not in love with—I had to focus my mind someplace else; otherwise, boredom would reign, and my attitude wouldn't be too hot, either. I decided to let my imagination run wild. I was no longer just another kid mowing a lawn in Baldwin, Long Island, but the starting center fielder at Shea Stadium. If I mowed around that corner in good time, I'd shag that fly ball before it went through the gap, or I'd take third on a hit-and-run. The Mets fans would be going nuts: "Go, Jake! Go, Jake! Mow! Mow! Mowwww!"

My fans were also there for me every time I cleaned my room, made a protein shake in the morning, or went for an after-school run. Whenever my energy flagged, I'd hear a roar go through the crowd, urging me on. It's amazing what happens when you tap into your imagination: you start to tap into your potential as well. I not only got my jobs done in better time and in better fashion, I also felt more connected to my future.

One day in that future I would give something back to those fans who supported me. My company worked with the National Football League to create its answer to baseball's seventh-inning stretch, called the "NFL fitness break," between the third and fourth quarters. At the Kansas City Chiefs' Arrowhead Stadium, I led eighty thousand football fans to the world's first NFL fitness break. Even with the home team down 17 points and it pouring rain, the fans joined in and roared so loudly that I wanted to strap on the pads myself! You wouldn't believe—but you will soon—the places your imagination can take you to in reality.

Are you ready to really go places? Your dreams can take you there if you let them. So if you're not a dreamer by now, it's time to become one—just don't stay in those clouds! I want you to keep those dreams lofty, but I also want you to come down to Earth and make them work for you every day. That's what I ask of my clients when they train with me, and that's what I want from, and for, you.

MUSCLE MAKER: *No Limits*

Do you think you can't develop washboard abs? Bulging biceps? Or fast legs? Nonsense! If you don't have these yet, it's because you haven't yet put your dreams to work! If you plug your ideas of what you want to become into my workout, you will achieve your dream shape.

Even some professional athletes haven't tested their limits, so do you think you've tested yours? Remember Dennis Rodman? At only 6 feet, 6 inches— small for a power forward—this wild-haired guy was the most extraordinary rebounder the NBA had ever seen, not simply because of his natural athletic ability, but because he took fitness to another level. After each game, in which he often played forty-plus minutes and would grab a dozen or often more boards, guess what he did for an encore? (No, I'm not talking about his penchant for late-night partying—that was for later.) He would jump right on an exercise bike and go full bore for thirty minutes. No wonder he never got tired!

Understand this: I'm not urging you to push it to Dennis's level (or to dye your head neon orange!). Instead, I want to use his example to show you what the human body is capable of if given the chance. Even if you start small, you can raise your intensity level and output a little bit each time you work out, as long as you stay consistent—and persistent.

Later in my workout you'll discover how to demand more from your body and how to get phenomenal results, all in a relatively short amount of time. For instance, we'll go way beyond the "Do one set of curls, then rest for a minute" approach. Your muscles aren't ready to rest yet! Your view of training will never be the same again.

▪ Power Tool—Use with Caution ▪

Your imagination is a powerful tool. Use it to propel you in the right direction, as it can be used in a wrong way as well—for example, thinking of all the reasons why you can't do something. Maybe you're nervous about a big game coming up and imagine a tragic blunder that could cost your team the game; or you paint a picture in your mind of the girl of your dreams laughing in your face when you finally muster up the courage to ask her out.

Always see your dreams in a positive light—and leave the nightmares for your unconscious in the middle of the night! Replace those pathetic images with winning ones, and when those situations arise, a much better scenario will play itself out. Remember, losers think of all the ways they can fail, while winners dream of all the routes to success. Losers look back on their failures as proof that they can't cut it, while winners look forward to all the things they can accomplish.

Do you think Steven Spielberg was tempted to hang it all up after a box-office bomb? Or that John Elway considered retiring after playing poorly in the Super Bowl? Forget it! Temporarily disappointed, they regrouped quickly and used these experiences to energize themselves even more in their quest for success. Then, after accomplishing their goals, they didn't stop there. They went about duplicating their successes—Wiels has had a string of hits, while Elway led his Denver Broncos to back-to-back Super Bowl victories.

What's their secret? It's simple: They both knew how to use their imagination by learning from failure while building on their successes.

Whether you recognize it or not, memories and past experiences make a huge impact on how you approach every day and every hurdle. Whether any given part of your past is positive or negative, it's bound to continue in exactly the same way until you do something different to alter its course. Even if something in your past is terribly negative, it doesn't foretell your future unless you allow it to.

▪ Activate Your Imagination! ▪

Somebody else might chide you for having an "overactive" imagination because you might have exaggerated just a bit about some situation. For example, "Yeah, my teacher told me that was the best essay he'd ever read and was considering letting me teach next week's classes." But I'll compliment you every time you exaggerate things—because it shows me where you want to go with that mind of yours.

Dreaming big is nothing to be ashamed of. Over the course of my life, my dreams and accomplishments have grown side by side—and that's not a coincidence! Dream small, and you will stay small.

What ultimately gave my dreams a kick start was lifting weights: the first time I lifted the curl bar in my basement, I felt totally empowered. Suddenly, I felt as if my dreams could become reality. It stuck in my mind: "If I can lift this ten times, I can do whatever I want to do." I did those ten reps and said, "Cool, I can reach those dreams. Now let's do fifteen." Then I was sore for a week!

My strength didn't happen overnight *physically,* but it did *mentally.* I knew that if I could make it through one of my tough workouts, I had what it took to follow any dream of mine. All the trouble I faced with my chubby body and stuttering speech I could now see myself overcoming. "Ten more minutes on the bike, one more pound of fat gone! Two more exercises, two more words I won't stumble over!" My imagination had *power,* just like that.

It's time to inject your imagination with power and believe in it. When you believe in what you're dreaming about, you'll put in 110 percent effort to snag those dreams.

▪ Seeing Is Believing ▪

Have you ever heard of visualization? It's certainly practiced and referred to by that name in the sports world, where everyone from quarterbacks to golfers visualizes what he wants to happen—whether a quarterback throwing a perfect spiral to his receiver cutting across the field or a golfer hitting a four-iron flush that fades right to the pin. Visualization techniques are used in many other arenas as well. Painters, architects, and filmmakers are celebrated "visual" artists, and chefs, carpenters, and mechanics use visualization in their work, too.

The best thing about visualization is that you, too, can use it and with just as much success as all those guys. It's free, it's easy, and it's fun! Try this: create a situation in your mind that you want to unfold in an exact way before you create it in life. You already visualize many times a day without being aware of it. When you clean your room, you have an idea of what it should look like when you're done—and your mom certainly does! Or you envision what might be on your history test and thus are better prepared when you take it the next day.

As you see, visualization can be an unconscious technique and still work for you. I'm asking you to make it conscious. Then you really can capture the visions you seek.

DREAM EXTREME: *If He Did It, I Can Too*

Let me tell you about some amazing feats: No one in major league base-ball had hit more than sixty home runs since Roger Maris hit sixty-one in 1961. It was one of those records that everyone thought would never be broken. Thirty-seven years later, in 1998, *two* players broke it: Mark McGwire of the St. Louis Cardinals and Sammy Sosa of the Chicago Cubs. The following year, the same two players hit more than sixty-one again!

To most, breaking this record just didn't seem possible—but people don't always take into account the amazing human spirit. While records such as this one seem almost impossible to beat, once an athlete (or athletes) actually does it, suddenly they appear well within the range of possibility. As far as McGwire and Sosa were concerned, each one realized that if the other could do it, he could too—twice!

Breaking the sound barrier also seemed to be an impossible dream. It just wasn't ever supposed to happen. But once it was broken by Chuck Yeager in 1947, countless other pilots did it in the following years!

What's the lesson here? It's this: No matter how extreme your dream, any-thing's possible if you believe in it. Anything that you seriously want in your life. Sink your mind into it first, then your teeth. You'll get there!

Before I aimed to flex my muscles onstage as a bodybuilder, I was always visualizing my muscles getting bigger—my chest growing with each bench press, my abs getting more defined with each sit-up. When I began serious training, my visualization went up another notch. I saw myself standing next to the giants of the sport—all those guys in the muscle mags I'd read about—and matching their muscles inch for inch. I'd nail every pose for the judges, nudg-ing aside my foes with a well-placed double-biceps pose.

Every muscle on my body was built up in my mind first, and these muscles were soon to follow the lead—well, except for my pesky calves! Do the same with yours, starting today. Visualize the attributes you want—leaping ability, a ripped physique, fast legs—and where you want to take them—to the basket-ball court, beach, soccer field. Keep your eyes on these prizes, and you're bound to do the work to seize them.

POWER HABIT: *Visualization*

Find a quiet place away from any distractions, then use this technique to have the success you've dreamed about.

1. Relax completely. Visualize what you want—maybe it's more muscles and better athletic performances or great grades and college scholarship offers; maybe it's being noticed by all the girls and getting *the* girl. Whatever it is, don't think of all the reasons why you can't have these things. Instead, *believe* that they will be yours.

2. Get over anything negative in your past—failures, bad experiences, self-doubt—that keeps you from achieving your dreams. Now you're a new guy who's not going to let those things slow you down anymore.

3. Paint the entire picture of your dream, including every detail. You'll then be prepared to live that dream.

4. Allow the sweet emotions of living that dream to flow through you. Remember the feeling those emotions give you so you can access them anytime you want when you're out there chasing your dream.

5. Map out how exactly to capture the success you want. What do you need to improve on? Do you need to shape up physically? Toughen up mentally? What do you need to add to your life? What needs to be subtracted?

6. Every morning before you get out of bed, visualize your dreams. Ask yourself what you need to do that day to get closer to them. Then determine how to make them come alive!

▪ Expand Your Field of Vision ▪

The best place to begin using visualization is in your training, as you imagine your body becoming strong, powerful, and muscular. Gold's Gym in Venice, California, where I often work out, is full of guys who do this. The most famous bodybuilding gym in the world, it's a place where the dreams of many of these fellas end up in creating the ultimate physique for themselves. Some have already achieved it.

But here's the rub: few of them achieve success in any other area. Many of them, in fact, barely have enough money to cover their gym membership and their supplements! I'm not saying that I've got it over all these people, but they could do so much more if they would simply expand their vision. Their scope is set on one target—their body—and therefore they miss out on success in other areas.

They've got the tools—they put them into practice every time they train— to improve many parts of their lives other than their body. All they need to do is call on their imagination to imagine more. And that's what I'm calling on you to do. With the help of this book, I want you to build the most impressive physique you ever thought possible, but I also want you to build an impressive future in other areas.

My late grandma Myra Duberstein, who played an enormous role in my life, used to have the same concern about me: too much tunnel vision. I'd spend all my free time lifting weights and reading muscle magazines. She'd shake her head. "Grandson, if you spent as much time reading quality books as you spent on your muscles, you'd be another Einstein!"

Does that sound familiar? Do you spend all your time focused on one area, such as sports? Does your Saturday play out like this: shooting hoops for hours, reading *Sports Illustrated,* logging on to espn.go.com, then making sure you don't miss the game on TNT that night? Expand your scope now, and you'll be thankful later.

REALITY CHECK: *Moving On to the Next Dream*

When I was fourteen, I was dead set on becoming the New York Knicks' next great power forward. One look at my six-foot-one height probably has you rolling your eyes and laughing your buttissimo off! But I believed it, and I was intent on putting the "power" into the forward position.

I never went on to make the Knicks' squad or even play in college, but my Knicks dreams pushed me further into the training world, where I belong. I've ended up doing things in this world that far outmatch the professional satisfaction I might have had as a Knick. So instead of dunking over Larry Bird back then, I'm trying to hop over fellow business competitors to the Fortune 500!

I had boundless energy and focused intently on my goals of becoming a Knick or a muscle man, but my grandma knew my goals were too limited.

Guess what? She was right, because as soon as I got rid of those limitations I began to achieve *truly* great things.

This point was driven home when I began training some of the most successful people in show business. For them, training to reach body perfection was certainly not the ultimate goal. Training made them feel and look great, but the most important thing it accomplished was to enable them to get ahead to the next level—in their careers, relationships, finances, education, you name it. What is your next level?

▪ The Wait Is Over! ▪

Are you ready to get into it? Are you getting pumped up? Anybody can hang back and talk, telling people what he's planning to do. Few, however, are willing to actually go out there and follow up on their words. If you train with me, I'll help make you better than your word!

I've never lifted weights just to lift weights. There had to be something more. So the first thing that popped into my head was Mr. America. I told myself, "If I'm going to do this, then I'm going for it. I'm not training just because I'm in the mood. The journey is great and all, but the prize is what I want." So winning the Mr. America competition became my mission. I never plotted it out on a timeline; instead, I just started to live it—through tenacious training and disciplined dieting.

I was no longer at the dreaming-it-up stage. I was now ready to take my dream up the mountain on my back. And that's what I've done with everything in my life. You can think of five thousand reasons why you shouldn't do something or can never succeed at it. But in the end the only person who will stop your success is you—because you didn't commit yourself to achieving it.

Don't wait until the ice-cream man starts to avoid your block because he feels guilty about how many Choco-Caramel Cream Bombs he's been selling you, or until you've smoked so many cigarettes that taking out the garbage makes you wheeze like an old man. I became sick and tired of stuttering my way through the school day and drowning my sorrows with a fast-food chowdown. I knew that route was a dead end.

Even if you don't catch yourself in time and you do get a serious scare because you haven't changed your ways—such as a drug overdose or being suspended from school for fighting—it's not too late. Some of my most motivated clients have been those who have hit rock bottom and made the decision never to set foot on that path again.

STUMBLING . . . TO SUCCESS: *Steven Spielberg Didn't Get into the Film School of His Choice?!*

You read that right, Mr. Movie himself wasn't admitted to the University of Southern California film school when he first applied—or later, when he re-applied. You can bet the school later regretted that decision! As a teenager, Wiels, as we all call him, faced other types of problems, such as his parents divorcing and being picked on regularly by bullies at school. But he had a powerful imagination that freed him, and he was committed to following that imagination.

That commitment is very apparent in every movie Spielberg makes, as every one of them—from *E.T.* to *Jurassic Park* to *A.I.: Artificial Intelligence*—displays an imaginary world unmatched by any other director. His imagination and commitment are the reasons his films have grossed more money than those of any other movie director. Following through on every last detail in his vision of imaginary worlds requires enormous willpower and energy, because production of a film can be tedious and last for a very long time.

From the start of his training, I was impressed by Wiels's ability to commit. This was a guy who hadn't worked out since junior high and wasn't exactly naturally endowed with muscle. But he wanted to change that, and once we started on his program, he stuck with it. He'd groan good-naturedly when I'd show up early to take him through the exercises at his home, but his fitness level went up at every workout. Now, before he sets out on a film shoot, he trains just as athletes do before their season begins. Weeks of long shooting days, deadline pressures, fattening craft services food, and little sleep turn many directors into chubby wrecks—but not Wiels!

Wiels was only six years old when his imagination first went wild. One day, while his three sisters and mother slept, his dad woke him up early to drive him into the dark desert a half hour outside Phoenix. They reached the rim of a canyon to which more than a hundred other parents and their children had journeyed. There he witnessed a spellbinding meteor shower that lit his imagination and much later inspired his breakthrough film, *Close Encounters of the Third Kind.* From that day forward, he kept that imagination lit, and millions of movie fans are grateful.

That same imagination helped him keep the bullies at school from beating up on him. How? By casting them in his early amateur movies. Now, rather than being shoved around by them, Wiels was ordering them where to walk, what to say, and how to say it! That's putting your imagination to great use!

Get with me now and commit. You'll no longer be waiting for things to happen to you or for the waves to crash down on you. You'll be riding on top of those waves, toward your goals. Once you make a serious commitment to a better lifestyle, starting with your body and mind, whatever you want will be yours.

BEFORE YOU LOOK AHEAD, LOOK IN THE MIRROR

TWO

I started my teenage years slowly, whether I was trying to pull off a stutter-free conversation or running the 50-yard dash in three days! No awards from the President's Council on Physical Fitness were coming my way anytime soon. However, I didn't cry myself to sleep every night. I still had plenty of friends, and I felt pretty good, considering how I looked in the mirror—partly because I never looked in the mirror!

It was pretty naive of me to think that I was a normal-looking teenager who was about to step into the good years—going out with girls, starring on the sport teams, starting to become a man. It never really occurred to me that I had a weight problem. My buddies loved to poke fun at my machine-gun delivery (you know, mmm-mm-my stut-stut-stut-terr-terring), but my extra flab was never a big deal. I was just a big guy, right? After all, they liked the same chocolate shakes and sacks of White Castle burgers that I did! Same story with my parents: I was just a big boy who liked his mom's chow!

I was overdue to make a crash landing into reality. It should have happened when my mom took me to buy my first suit for my bar mitzvah. I was thirteen years old and primed to let the girls check out the sharp-dressed man. Mom took me to Syms clothing store on Long Island. The salesman sized me up in about three seconds, and then he led me and my mom past all the racks of nice-looking suits for regular kids to the "Husky" section.

I was pretty flattered, thinking this section was for the strong, athletic guys.

That was when the salesman yanked out a blue suit that could have subbed for a shower curtain, with buttons. One sleeve bore the distinguished label "Husky," neatly embroidered on two inches of ribbon.

Just to double-check that this label should be worn with pride, I asked my mom, "What does that mean?"

"It means you are a young man now," said the best actress in the world, my mom.

Yes sir! Just what I thought; I was becoming a man, and this proved it. I was so convinced of this honor that I wanted to wear this label like a colonel wears his stripes. I was ready to march into my bar mitzvah with my "Husky" label in full view until my mom convinced me that it wasn't appropriate for such an occasion. I didn't give up without a fight, however—she had to promise me a month's worth of allowance in advance first!

There was no crash landing into reality that time. I was happy, cruising along in the fantasy lane that went nowhere. Little did I know it then, but I was about to enter a world in which reality would hit me smack in the face. A place where everything was a bigger deal—talking to girls, playing on the team, talking in class. Yeah, I'm talking about high school, where the standard was higher for whatever you did and where suddenly not everyone was friends anymore.

I wasn't ready because I was afraid to get naked—both physically and mentally—and really look at myself. That would have taken courage that I hadn't mustered yet. What about you? Where are you in this process? Have you ever stood in front of a mirror and really looked at yourself? Not just at how you look, but how you act, how you think, how you dream?

With this book in your hands, I want you to ask yourself these questions. I want you to get to the bottom of who you are. Only then can you get to the business of turning the negatives—in your person, your physique, and your life—into positives.

Those guys who automatically get the best-looking girl, who are handed the starting job as quarterback, who get top grades without cracking a book? Don't envy them. Often they don't know who they are or what they want until years later. You may even find yourself at a class reunion one day, the object of those guys' envy!

▪ Wake-up Call Number One ▪

When I was a teenager, my alarm clock often had to go off twice before I got my buttissimo out of bed. I wasn't ready to face the day yet. I also wasn't ready to face myself and truly acknowledge the stuttering lump that I'd become. It was a lot easier to hide under the covers!

All that changed when I received a couple of serious wake-up calls—the first from the outside world, the second from inside myself. Unlike my experience at Syms, I wasn't going to sleep through these!

I needed something big to wake me from my stupor, something to strike me right in the heart because it would involve something I loved—which perhaps my brain would notice! That was basketball, a great love of mine since I was little. Whether beating my younger brothers down at the park or watching my New York Knicks, it was in my blood.

When eighth-grade tryouts were announced, I was excited: finally, I'd have a chance to show off my patented drop step, à la Willis Reed, which I'd added to my game after seventh grade. I hadn't spent much time honing it, but I was sure that with my big body, it would be easy. I had a good feeling: this year I was going to see more playing time than pining time.

I went through the week of tryouts picking my spots—getting a rebound here, throwing up a hook shot there. I didn't play very hard because I knew I was already on the team. Then the roster listing the guys who had made the cut was posted in the gym. I walked over with my buddies to check it out, already dueling with them over who was going to see the ball the most that year.

My eyes landed on the page and immediately my buddies' names jumped out at me, but mine was nowhere to be found. There had to be an explanation, so I ripped the roster off the wall to see if my name was on the other side. No dice. Have you ever been punched in the gut without expecting it? That's how I felt.

Truth is, I gave myself that punch. It was a self-inflicted wound, and it hurt worse than anything I'd experienced in my young life. The small amount of confidence that I did have was built on my supposed athletic ability, and now I couldn't even make the team? I didn't even look at my buddies as I made a beeline for the nearest exit. How was I ever going to show my face to them again? Or to my little brothers, who had bought into every one of my athletic boasts?

I felt as if I had lost my safety net; I was free-falling into the pit of despair.

Everybody saw it, but no one could help me climb out—until a clever girl who lived down the street gave me a poem that snapped me out of it in a hurry. In fact, it changed my entire life. I hadn't read many poems up until that point (or afterward!), but this one was perfectly crafted for me and came at the perfect time. It's called "Don't Quit" and has words that I live by to this day. Here's the first stanza (I'll save the next two for later in the book!):

DON'T QUIT POEM: *Down but Not Out!*

When things go wrong, as they sometimes will,
When the road you're trudging seems all uphill,
When the funds are low and the debts are high,
And you want to smile, but you have to sigh,
When care is pressing you down a bit,
Rest, if you must, but don't you quit.

I immediately memorized this poem. It was only words—just like this book you're reading—but it was the best gift I'd ever received (I hope *Get Strong!* ranks up there for you, too!). I recited it to my family at dinnertime that evening. My father was surprised by my ability to memorize it so quickly. Even more, though, he was impressed by my strong will to follow the poem's meaning. He told me, "Jake, son, if you're so determined to make the team, I'm going to help you."

He did, by week's end. Using the thick cardboard underside of my old train set, he concocted a backboard. Then he nailed on a rusty iron hoop that was lying around in the basement. As you can tell, we weren't rolling in dough, but this "basket" meant more to me than any brand-spanking-new getup that my buddies from the ritzier part of town had their dads get for them. My father put time and effort into my dream, and I was ready to make him proud. Suddenly, I spent every waking moment in front of that hoop while my two little brothers rebounded for me—no matter what the weather. I recall many cold, snowy days when I played until my left hand felt as if it was going to freeze off—you didn't expect me to wear a glove on my shooting hand, did you?—and late nights under the backyard lamp, playing until my mom begged me (and my brothers, if they were still out there with me!) to come inside.

I knew I had nobody to blame for not making the team but myself. I wanted to make sure that scenario never repeated itself. It didn't. I made the team the next year. I was on my way to basketball stardom—or was I?

▪ Wake-up Call Number Two ▪

Actually, I haven't told you the whole story. Yes, my basketball skills improved as I got maximum usage out of what my dad had made for me, and that helped me get onto the team. However, I wasn't starting on the team and was by no means a star! See, what I neglected to tell you is that my dad bought me something else that didn't see as much action: a brand-new weight set—which promptly started to rust, sitting unused in the backyard. You heard it right: at fourteen, Mr. Fitness took a pass on weight training.

Soon after he bought the set, my dad called me out to the backyard. He noticed I hadn't picked up a weight since it had appeared on the Steinfeld property. "I've got a great idea. Let's do some bench presses," he said. With a fresh pack of Twinkies and the Mets game waiting for me in the TV room, it sounded like an awful idea. "No thanks, Dad," I said. Though he'd been in the U.S. Navy and wasn't to be messed with, he was ultimately a softie. He asked you to do something only once; it was up to me to follow through. I realize now, looking back, that he was teaching me that I had to take responsibility for my own life.

He could provide the tools and the support, but it was up to me to use them to make myself better at whatever I wanted to do. And, as any good basketball player will tell you, there's a lot more to the game than any one thing, including shooting baskets! There's also the small matter of being in good shape. For every hour I had spent outside hooping it up, I'd eaten an extra cookie or slice of pizza. Shooting baskets had become my license to pig out on a daily basis. So while I'd spent plenty of time developing a nice touch around the basket, I sure didn't look any different! This fact didn't exactly raise my chances of dominating on the basketball team, except at the pregame dinners!

Before my sophomore season, however, my second wake-up call came. It was my rediscovery of those weights, now sitting unused on the laundry shelf (my dad had made me move them from the backyard, since it didn't look as if they'd ever be used). While the first wake-up call had forced me to open my eyes, this one made me jump out of bed! More significantly, it had me turn my eyes to the mirror—where I really saw myself for the first time.

What I saw there wasn't a pretty picture: my stomach rolled over my belt; I had two chins; my round arms didn't show even a hint of muscle definition. Oddly, though, all this didn't depress me because I knew I was through conning myself into believing that I was a great athlete. I was a tub—but was that the end of the story? No way, buddy, it was only the beginning, now that I was finally standing up to *myself* and facing my problems square on. In fact, I now viewed these so-called problems as challenges, and I was getting pumped up about taking them on! My vision of fifty thousand Madison Square Garden fans cheering just for me certainly helped, but the biggest pump—for both my muscles *and* my mind—came from simply lifting the curl bar.

REALITY CHECK: *Ringing the Big Bell*

Each round of a boxing match commences with a ringing bell. In such a brutal sport, "answering the bell" every round is the mark of a tough competitor who's ready to keep slugging away. That describes me pretty well—because ever since those two early alarm bells, I've answered every one that was meant for me. It's a great habit to develop, since it shows the world that you're prepared for whatever challenges come your way. Coach expects you to show up the first day of practice in good shape? You show up in great shape! Your classmates pick you to be class president because you promised one party per month? You deliver!

Eventually you'll reach a point where you're the one ringing the bells that other people have to answer! As a deal maker, I now use it as one of my common practices. For instance, when I launched Major League Lacrosse, I took some stars from the various teams to the New York Stock Exchange. Once there, we looked over the trading floor, then I got to ring the bell that signified the close of trading. Now, that's a feeling of power!

That big bell also signified a lot of firsts: my first time visiting Wall Street, my first season of Major League Lacrosse, and the first time I wore a suit on TV! (By the way, unlike my first shower-curtain-with-buttons suit, this one was custom-made!)

▪ Wide Awake at Last! ▪

After that second wake-up call, I was awake as never before. Staring at my reflection in the mirror while I did rep after rep, I simultaneously saw who I had been and who I was going to become. To an observer, it might have seemed as if I had a lot of work in front of me. In my mind, however, it was only a matter of time, because I felt empowered to go after my goals.

I still looked like the old chubby, stuttering Jake, but in some key respects, I had changed. After I answered that second alarm bell, the insecurity, laziness, and uncertainty that had dominated my past didn't have a place to hang out any longer. I had achieved a clear understanding of what it took to get to a new and improved present and future. My discovery of training and its inherent power changed everything for the better.

Weight training gave me the control over my life that I had been lacking. The weights made me feel much more powerful and energetic than shooting baskets ever had. There was no way I was going to give them up! Soon, as my muscles and confidence grew, both my stuttering and my stuff-my-face tendency began to dwindle.

Training with weights helped me on the basketball court, too. No longer content with just making the team, I became team captain and starter all through high school. My new rock-hard physique made my opponents wince and my coach smile.

Ever since then, I've been grateful whenever I get another wake-up call, because it alerts me to what's lacking in the present and how exactly I can improve my future. The same holds true for you.

Think about it for a minute: What kind of wake-up calls have you had? Maybe your coach thinks you'd make a better mascot than middle linebacker or your mother was pleasantly surprised when the restaurant rehired you this summer—as dishwasher. Those are big alarm clocks, buddy! How did you react? Rather than ignoring them and drifting further away from what you can become, I encourage you to use them to push you toward reaching your potential.

▪ Ask the Tough Questions . . . of Yourself! ▪

As you've seen, back then I took a pretty unflinching look at myself. Now it's your turn. Take a good long look in a mirror. If that makes you uneasy, I'm thrilled! You're looking at yourself honestly. If you truly want to improve yourself, it's crucial that you examine what it is about you that needs work. The physical shortcomings will probably leap out at you first—maybe a flabby midsection, stick-thin legs, or no-show biceps. However, I'm more interested in how you feel and think right now. Change the inside before the outside, and success will come much more quickly—in both camps!

Are you happy with your life right now? Do you think you're headed in a positive direction? What challenges are you meeting well? Are there any that are getting the better of you? How do you view yourself? Do others look at you the same way? If there's a difference, why? Of the character traits that you don't like, why do you think they exist? Has each trait improved or gotten worse over time?

If you feel as if you are perpetually having to prove yourself, maybe it's because you doubt your own abilities. If you are easily annoyed by people or things, perhaps you are always irritable. If you sense that you can never satisfy other people, the truth might be that you rarely satisfy yourself!

Few guys are brave enough—and patient enough—to answer these questions or face their conclusions. Just like a good medical checkup, only if you know what ails you can you get better. You must reckon with exactly who you are right now, for better or worse. Then you will know exactly what you need to work on. If you're struggling with seeing exactly who you are or think there are some problematic elements in you that you may not be consciously aware of, ask a good friend who is willing to answer questions about you in a frank way. Just don't get angry at him or her afterward if the answers are more brutal than you'd like—they're supposed to help!

Most people want to be told only how great they are—how funny, smart, and good-looking. That, however, prevents growth. If you want to reach your full potential, you need to listen to criticism and perhaps even seek it out. You have to be able to like that person you see in the mirror. No matter how many flaws you (or your pal) detect or how low you've sunk, only if you are kind to yourself will life do you any favors!

So please don't beat yourself up anymore. The game has not even begun for you. You're still in the on-deck circle. By the time you get to the plate, armed with my workout training and helpful thoughts, you will be able to hit one out of the park almost every time! To do that, you must feel good about yourself, because when you do, others will feel good about you as well. All the successful people I have trained in Hollywood are comfortable with themselves, and this is one of their many secrets of their success. After all, how can you expect other people to appreciate you unless you do?

Before I looked in the mirror, I wasn't exactly on a hot streak. My fortunes with sports, girls, and schoolwork were all heading south. Starting to train, however, reversed these fortunes by 180 degrees. I didn't strike gold in all these things instantly, but success was ensured because I had begun to tackle each problem area of my life. Behind my stuttering self was a smooth, powerful talker; inside my round, underachieving body was a muscular athlete. I was just waiting to emerge! I had serious potential, and weight training brought it out.

DREAM EXTREME: *Pounce on the Potential*

The word "potential" is thrown around a lot. Maybe it's been applied by others to you and to your ability to study, play a sport, or be a mature person. Sometimes it is used in a slightly negative sense, so that the statement "You have potential" expresses the opinion that you'll never fulfill it. It's used after the fact to describe an unfortunate scenario, such as "It's too bad about Joe Bean. He had so much potential."

The person who knows best what you are capable of, however, is you—no matter what anybody else says about you. Even if you are written off by someone who thinks you'll never fulfill your promise, it's up to you to prove that person wrong.

A lot of people who knew me when I was growing up didn't think I'd amount to much. They certainly didn't predict that I would become a successful entrepreneur, "trainer to the stars," founder of a professional sports league, and so on. Heck, they didn't even see me as team captain on the basketball team. But if I'd listened to them, I wouldn't be able to list any of those accomplishments.

Your potential is in your hands. No matter how great a father and mother you have, how smart a teacher, how skilled a coach, nobody can tap your potential the way you can. Soaking up all of their wisdom and encouragement will help, but ultimately you are the master of your own potential. When I picked up that very first weight, it was a moment that I'll never forget. I suddenly felt the surge of potential from within. I saw muscles, a beautiful woman (who turned out to be my wife, Tracey!), financial success, happiness—all within range.

The same can happen to you. You too will notice that your potential is truly unlimited if you let your imagination roam and put plenty of work and know-how behind it. There's a tremendous satisfaction that comes from knowing that you do everything you can to maximize your potential in everything you try. What's more, you'll have no regrets!

▪ Don't Be Someone You're Not, Especially Mike Stein ▪

When I started the Body by Jake business, I didn't have an agent to approach potential clients about endorsements and product licensing. I had built up a good name because of the media attention I received from training my celebrity clients, but that was about it. This meant that I had to pitch potential clients myself.

Every day, I'd sit down to read a sports marketing paper, on the lookout for an endorsement deal. I came across a company based in Lubbock, Texas, called USA Wet, that was making a sports drink to rival Gatorade. Without much forethought, I dialed it up. Beside the phone lay another article I'd read that morning; it was from *The Hollywood Reporter* and was all about how agents were the only way to seal a deal. Therefore, while the phone rang at the other end, I decided that this company must not find out that I didn't have an agent.

When the secretary answered, I introduced myself—as Mike Stein. You know, the agent for Jake Steinfeld and Body by Jake, Inc.! I lowered my voice a few notches and cranked up the New York accent. I'd done many prank calls on friends, but this was a first in a professional setting (and I'm not necessarily recommending this approach!).

Apparently my act was pretty well honed, because not only did the secretary put me through to the president, Big John, but Big John liked the idea so much he told me—er . . . Mike Stein—to fly down to Texas that week. Gulp. In a panic, I agreed.

Then I had another harebrained idea. What about my attorney, Bob Lieberman, going as Mike Stein? Bob rightly declined, saying "I'll go as Bob, thanks."

Needless to say, Big John was disappointed that Mike didn't show up and wouldn't sign on the dotted line until he met him face to face.

He said to Bob, "Ol' Mike and I just hit it off. How about I fly to L.A. next week and meet with you, Jake, and Mike, and we'll all have dinner together and make a deal?"

Now I was really worried. Bob and I agreed to meet Big John at the Palm Restaurant on Santa Monica Boulevard for lunch. When he arrived, he shook our hands and then, of course, asked where Mike was. Bob kicked me under the table.

"Uh, he's on location doing some work in Hawaii and sends his regards," I said. Sweat was pouring down my forehead, and my act was rapidly falling apart.

Big John looked at me carefully. "Jake, you sound a lot like ol' Mike," he accused.

"We grew up together on Long Island," I spat out.

Big John raised his eyebrows. He was no dummy. "Listen, Jake, I want to meet Mike Stein before this deal gets done. We really connected on the phone. You call me when Mike gets back to town, and he and I will put this deal together. I'll be seeing you," said Big John and left, leaving a perfectly good steak untouched on the table.

As you probably guessed, that deal never got done. It's an extreme example of how not being yourself can sink your ship before it leaves the harbor. If I'd been myself, my business would have been off to a flying start. Instead, I was left kicking myself (in the same spot Bob had, figuratively speaking!) about the missed opportunity.

Popular culture saturates you with images of people you're supposed to want to be like, from musicians to actors to sports stars. You're told to wear Kobe Bryant's shoes and watch the Farrelly brothers' movies. In an Eminem video, "The Real Slim Shady," he pokes fun at this marketing phenomenon, with a roomful of young men looking just like him in white T-shirts, jeans, and a bleached-blond crew cut. When you look around your high school and see how similarly people dress and style themselves, you realize it's not that much of a stretch.

I dare you to be different. There's only one Eminem, only one Kobe Bryant, so you've got to be you. Trust yourself and go your own way.

TRAINING TRIP-UPS: *The Chucklehead Syndrome*

For those guys who want to get big fast, be on guard about this. You will see it mostly among aspiring young bodybuilders, but it has also been spotted among the mainstream gym crowd. Muscleheads are who I call chuckleheads: guys who think and talk about muscle to the point that their brains become about as bright as their biceps! Chucklehead syndrome is worse; it occurs when guys are driven to build muscle obsessively in the belief that they look too thin.

It's often characterized by a particular pattern in which a guy starts making gains, which lead him to compare himself to others in the gym, at school, or in magazines. Invariably he comes across someone who's bigger and stronger, which results in his questioning his physique and, in a gross distortion of body image, considering himself to be way too small (even though he may, in fact, be more muscle-bound than The Rock!). At that point he starts doubting everything: his training, his diet, his supplementation, even his potential!

I used to love to compare my expanding muscles to those of the fellas in the magazine pages, but in my mind it was healthy competition. I encourage the same healthy approach for you, in which you keep some perspective about how big you can become and are patient with your progress. Size is not everything! When was the last time the most muscular guy on your team was the best player? Or had the most dates? Almost never.

Instead, concentrate on the great things you can do with your body besides simply slapping on muscle. Make those muscles usable—in sport or in life. The MQ (Muscle Quotient) test that you will take later measures what your muscles are capable of, but not their size. Not everyone is going to be a muscle man or dunk a basketball. Feel good about who you are and appreciate the gifts you have!

▪ One Thing Leads to Many Others ▪

It's well known that a good education opens worlds for you, but did you know that training does the same? Training put into motion everything in my life that wouldn't budge—my weight problem, stuttering, bad grades, and failure with girls. I quickly knew that great things were around the corner. First I felt and saw my muscles grow as my fat disappeared; then people began to treat me differently. The self-confidence that had eluded me for so long was now a part of me.

Amazingly, once I got on top of the training, everything else began to improve, while all the hard work I put into workouts made everything else easier to deal with. Getting up in the morning, walking down the school hallway holding my head up, outdueling my competitors in my chosen sport—in all these areas, I experienced tremendous progress. The fact that eventually I could switch from the baggy shirts that used to camouflage my round body to form-fitting ones illustrates perfectly just how far I had come.

In very little time, people started to notice that I was no longer that chubby Jake who couldn't be taken seriously. I'll never forget the first comment I got about my new physique, when one of the guys told me, "Yo, Jake, what's with the biceps, man? You been workin' out or whaat?" Topping that was a girl who touched my arm and said, "Ohhh, Jake, you've got muscles!" I was already motivated, but these positive reinforcements fueled me even further. You, too, will receive many compliments after you begin to make some impressive changes—and if you're like I was and never had heard these sorts of compliments before, they'll make you prouder than you've been in a long time, maybe ever!

Before long, I had an image that I wanted to maintain, and even build on—and make my previous bloated image history! Every night in my basement, I chipped away at my fat and added a little more muscle. It was what I looked forward to most each day. Becoming stronger and more muscular became my passion—one that has never died! I couldn't get enough of anything in the media that had to do with it, from the Hercules movies to the bodybuilding magazines.

I don't know how training will change *you*, but there's no doubt that it will. Wait until you see what happens! You'll bring this new sense of power over your life to everything you do, and then you'll realize that you have the power to alter whatever you choose. Training will put you into the driver's seat of your life.

▪ Get Naked! ▪

I'm talking about getting naked in both respects—mental and physical—when you begin to train. Dig up all your weaknesses and problems while you work out and, one by one, wipe them away as you push your body with the weights. Training has a way of stripping you to the core, if it's done right. It's funny: you walk out of a workout feeling completely relaxed and refreshed—even though you're pumped and sweaty!

Once you start to feel good about yourself, everybody else will feel good about you, too: your parents, brothers and sisters, friends, teachers, coaches. You'll probably thump your forehead and ask yourself, "Why didn't I do this earlier!" Why? Because you refused to get naked!

There are so many reasons why: being glued to the tube or stuck on the Web for hours every day; family members who view exercise as an expression of mania; friends who can't be dragged to the gym, yet are game for a cigarette anytime; your own problem with drugs or alcohol; the misconception that working out is just for jocks; the idea that preparing for college and life is only about hitting the books; the belief that training requires tons of time.

I challenge you to put down the remote control, the mouse, and the phone, and start heaving some weights. You'll still have time to press and double-click, but now your time will be more focused. I challenge you to put down the French fries and soda, and instead, eat and drink what will make you strong. (Don't worry, you'll see in Chapter 9 that one day a week you can eat whatever you choose!) I challenge you to drop the attitude that will keep you away from your workouts and to substitute an attitude of excitement with which to greet every training session.

▪ There's Only One Way to Think: Positively! ▪

There are many dominant players in sports today, but few remain top dog year after year. Michael Jordan dominated from the moment he stepped onto an NBA floor and went on to record the highest scoring average (31.5 points per game for the Chicago Bulls) of any player in NBA history. Jordan was known best for his phenomenal athletic skills and second-to-none killer instinct. However, his most impressive weapon of all was his ability always to think positively no matter what hurdle he faced. In a sport where so many games are won or lost in the last few minutes, he always came through in the clutch.

Jordan first showed this remarkable trait back when he was your age, after he got cut from his high school varsity basketball team. Yes, Air Jordan himself. Two years later, he ranked as one of the top high school players in the country. In his early NBA years, people labeled him as only a scorer who couldn't play defense or make his teammates better. He answered by leading the Bulls to three straight NBA championships and made the all-defensive team each year.

Jordan then lost his father in a tragic murder, and later the media leveled charges that he was a compulsive gambler. This turmoil, combined with his feeling that he had little left to prove on the court, pushed him into an early retirement in which he flirted with professional baseball—where again the media hounded him, this time even questioning his athletic skills.

A year and a half later, Michael returned to the NBA, ready to turn all these negatives into positives. In his first year back, he played erratically and ended the season on a very uncharacteristic note—turning the ball over in the final minute of a playoff game, costing his team the game. Sorely disappointed, Jordan regained his optimism in time to announce to the assembled press how much better he'd be next year. True to his word, he was, leading the Bulls to another stunning three-peat and retiring as King of the Mountain. What's more, Michael—four years later, at age thirty-eight—is returning to the game, which is now dominated by twentysomethings. That's thinking positively!

Maybe I'm not about to try to play midfielder for one of my MLL teams, but I take the same attitude into my workouts. When I'm doing push-ups, I mentally go through what I need to accomplish that day. By the time I've finished with my workout, not only have I worked my body, but I've also mentally conducted a meeting, made phone calls, had a successful business lunch, approved a proposal, and then greeted my great family at the end of the day! I know the outcome of every one of my daily events before I start my workday—and each of those outcomes is a positive one, believe me!

If you want to make the most of your opportunities, you, too, should become a positive thinker—in every part of your day, including your workouts. Many negative thinkers don't even notice opportunities! Thinking negatively only slows you down, but thinking positively puts you into overdrive. When an obstacle comes into your way, you think of a way to overcome it rather than worrying about how it can squash you. Positive people rebound from every disappointment rather than remaining disappointed.

Positive thinking puts your psyche into the future and all the great things you'll accomplish, but negative thinking only reminds you of your past failures and traps you in the present. Maybe you want to be a great surfer, filmmaker, lawyer; the first waves, shooting problems, or cases you encounter will probably leave you scratching your head. If you keep at it, however, and remind yourself that everyone struggles in the beginning, you will be performing well before too long.

Positivity and negativity draw a crowd in equal measure. If you're the first to offer an opinion about a new kid in school, plenty of others will second your assessment, whether it's positive or negative. Likewise, how you describe a painting you've done before you show it off to family and friends will affect its reception. Which attitude do you want to evoke?

I want you to greet each day as if it's going to be a great one, rain or shine, rather than focusing on the clouds and heading back to bed. Negativity kills dreams in their tracks. Positivity keeps your dreams alive until they become reality!

▪ Bring Out the BMOC Inside You! ▪

It's time for you to become the BMOC—you know, Big Man On Campus. Yep, I'm talking to you, even if you're less than six feet tall and weigh barely over a buck forty. By the end of this book, you'll know what it takes to be a BMOC wherever you go, from high school to college and beyond. If you want to be big, you can become big. Even if you don't, you'll become big in other ways if you follow my lead.

I've trained plenty of BMOCs who could barely pull off a pull-up but exhibited all the characteristics of leaders who stockpiled successes like a musclehead stockpiles muscles. Technically, I was the trainer of these powerful men in the entertainment field (and I pushed many of them to be able to squeeze a dozen or so pull-ups, by the way!), but they also trained me in ways that extended into every area of my life, ways I can't wait to share with you.

STUMBLING . . . TO SUCCESS: *Harrison Ford Had No Idea Indiana Jones Was Inside Him*

Harrison Ford, or "the H-Man," as I call him, is a true BMOC. While wielding as much power as any actor in the biz, he is never pretentious. In fact, you wouldn't even know he was a movie star if you met him on the street. When he was younger, he certainly didn't know it. He got expelled from a college in Wisconsin, then made his way to California to try acting. The floodgates didn't exactly open, so, being the determined guy that I know so well (on an off day, he sometimes tired *me* out in the gym!), he decided to find another way to support his young family.

He decided on carpentry, which he learned by reading every book on the subject at his local library! In a short time, Harrison started getting work from many people in the entertainment industry—as a carpenter. It wasn't what he had envisioned when he first moved to L.A., but it more than paid the bills. It became a comfortable living, and for a while he forgot that he had even been an actor. He now looked in the mirror and saw only a carpenter. But deep within him the fire to showcase his acting talent still burned. Do you think it was an accident that he was a carpenter for many people in the film industry? No way, buddy!

One day, fortune smiled on Harrison in a once-in-a-lifetime way. He was working on the office of a certain filmmaker named George Lucas, who had given Harrison a bit part in his first film, *American Graffiti,* four years before. George was going through the first *Star Wars* script with a couple of his assistants and wanted to hear a character's part read out loud. He asked this former-actor now-carpenter guy working outside his door to read the lines of Han Solo. As they say, the rest is history.

I hope you're beginning to see who you are and what you can become. Every talent and ambition that you have will come out of hiding—and you'll capitalize on your vast potential. You, the BMOC, will not only enter into arenas where you want to be, you will stay and dominate them as well! It won't be easy, but we're going to take the process step by step. Be consistent, and I know you'll get there.

THE POWER IS THERE—IT'S
TIME TO TURN IT ON!

You've checked yourself out in the mirror and have a pretty good idea about how you'd like to improve the outside, as well as the inside. Now you're probably itching to start! Before you leap ahead into my workout, though, take a few more minutes and check under your hood. What's there?

Excuse the car analogy, but L.A. is all about what you drive, just as it's about what you look like. Among the truly successful, however, what you have going on under your hood and in your head is what really counts! To dominate on L.A.'s crowded highways and in its hypercompetitive industries, you've got to have a serious engine.

Your high school probably doesn't look that much different, with its crowded hallways and plenty of competition to see who will reach the top. If you're not there yet, you will be. Why? Because you already have an engine inside you that's bursting with potential! You just need to start it up first.

You probably dream about being the BMOC in three main areas: with the girls, on the sports team, and in the classroom. To get those coveted spots—in that cute girl's heart, on the starting backfield, or in Princeton's incoming class—you need a jacked-up engine with stamina, toughness, and awesome power. Once we get that twelve-cylinder humming, you can catch up to whatever you've set your sights on. With my training, you'll suddenly see that *everything* you want is within reach.

Together, we're going to bring that big-time engine of yours out of the garage and drive to some extraordinary places. But there are several things that you'll have to do first.

▪ Zooming Past the Problems ▪

You're in a boxing match. In one corner is you, and in the other corner? You! If you truly want the things we've been talking about, it's time to say good-bye to the old you. No matter how out of shape you are, how poor your MQ or SAT scores are, how long it's been since you've had a date, whatever it is—it's all in the past. After all, you haven't taken that 550 Maranello Ferrari that is yourself out for a spin yet.

I've met some very impressive people in my time, many of whom had grown up in pretty difficult circumstances—with divorced parents, poverty, violence—but ultimately the biggest thing standing in the way of their success was themselves.

STUMBLING . . . TO SUCCESS:
Too Revved Up to Go Up

One of my friends is a Hollywood stuntman. Early on, he struggled to find work despite his considerable talent, and he really didn't know how to improve things. To others, however, it was obvious: He'd have to get rid of his nasty temper! The fact that he didn't listen very well, either, didn't help his cause. Fortunately, I had his ear—and his muscles. As we steadily accelerated our training pace at each workout, he began to focus on reducing his anger and eliminating his outbursts.

One day after training, we sat down and talked about his challenges. I told him that he was one of the top stuntmen in the business, but that something within him was keeping him from showcasing his talent and earning a good living.

He wasn't ready to accept that, however, and started playing the blame game. (By the way, in the blame game everybody loses, so that's one competition you can stay away from!) I distracted him by suggesting that maybe something in his past still angered him. He nodded his head and was silent. Then he finally began to tell me something that he'd held in for a long, long time. Some brutal things had happened to him during his upbringing. People he had trusted had ended up betraying and disappointing him, and so he expected the same treatment from just about everyone he came across—especially if he was in a position of authority. His tough family background had created a lot of internal anger that did not need much provocation to come out.

I asked him if he wanted to put an end to this self-destructive cycle, and he gave me the same look he gave me whenever I challenged him to do another set of curls. In other words, *yes!* We began working, step by step, on how to approach the world in a healthier, more positive way. Before he went for his next job, I had him change how he presented himself. We tried to replace his trademark anger and hostility with openness and calm. He was suspicious that it wouldn't work because he had tried "faking it" before and felt like a "phony." No wonder—a so-called phony has a mismatched inside and outside. It was time to get them on the same page, and the right page!

Dealing with his past helped him to feel better inside. This talented guy had always possessed an impressive engine, but it had often gone out of control. Now he knew why, and his new self-awareness improved both his behavior and his future. He got the very next stunt job he applied for! Today he is one of the most successful stuntmen in the business.

You see something similar to my stuntman buddy's case all the time with some young guys. Their rocky relationship with their parents spills out all over the place. A guy like that might dislike the way his father speaks to him, and then he imagines that he hears the same tone of voice from every coach he has. He constantly argues with his mother and then does the same with his teachers.

If that describes you, recognize that even if your relationship with your parent or parents is rocky, it doesn't have to damage every other relationship you have with someone in authority. Let me tell you this, though: No one wins when you don't get along with your parents. Maybe it's the result of a single thing that they did or you did; maybe it's the result of many things and goes back a long way. Whatever it is, tell yourself right now that you're going to repair your relationship. The best way to do that is through respect. No matter what's happened in your shared past, there are very few parents who don't deserve respect. After all, they've raised you and they love you (even if you don't believe it sometimes!). You might not be at the receiving end of that respect yet, depending on what's occurred in the past, but if you continue to respect and love your parent(s), it will soon go both ways!

Do you have other struggles that have you down? For me, putting on size "husky" pants or shrinking from view whenever my teacher asked if somebody would read a passage aloud was depressing. I knew I didn't want that to be my life! Will your struggles be your life? No way! We're going to solve your problems together. Keep reading.

Do you react to others around you in a way that benefits both them and you? Do you respond to challenging situations by facing them with optimism and preparedness? My stuntman pal didn't, and he learned that he was flushing his life down the toilet because he had been unwilling to take a hard look at himself. After some serious soul-searching, he made a decision to change.

That's what I'm asking you to do: to decide to change—not just to make a wish that this or that were better, but to make a decision. A wish is useless until you follow it up by your decision that your struggles will cease and your victories increase! Remember, *a wish changes nothing, but a decision changes everything.*

When I was young, I had a strong wish to become a guy worth taking notice of—whether on the playing field, strolling down the beach, or speaking in front of a crowd. However, nothing I was then resembled that wish, unless you count my ability to slam Devil Dogs down my throat! Weight training put my wishes into action. While my problems with my weight and my stuttering didn't disappear instantly, I now believed that they would over time. I had made a decision to get strong and gain control—it was the best decision I'd ever made!

Down in my basement alone, it was just me and my weights. The only way I wouldn't get a great workout would be if I didn't put in the effort myself. I decided then and there that I wouldn't let the weights beat me. I would be the boss. These weights were going to work for me, building the muscle and confidence I had been missing for so long, every time I trained. I started to believe that I was powerful, and guess what? I *became* powerful! If you believe, you will achieve. That is what this book is all about.

▪ Keys to Your 550 Maranello Ferrari ▪

Believe it or not, you've got a V-12 Maranello in there—not a Viper or even an Escalade, but the big daddy! Yeah, I'm talking to you. Maybe, before you picked up this book, you worried that you might not make the team or the grade this year. Don't, because everything you need—the stamina, toughness, and power that characterize a V-12—can be developed with focus and dedication.

I need you to agree to work out with me at least three to four times a week. Follow up on that promise on a weekly basis, and you'll have those attributes in abundance. Once you start to see your V-12 in action, your belief in yourself will skyrocket. When something extraordinary happens, such as scoring an improbable goal in the final seconds of a game or the best-looking girl in your class giving you the eye, you won't quite believe it at first. But if you believe that you're capable of such feats, they'll start happening all the time!

Before I ever received the set of keys to my first car—and before I had any clue that I had an engine of my own to reckon with—my father gave me a different kind of set . . . *of weights*. This bare-bones weight set gave me more freedom and power than any souped-up Trans Am. They allowed me to find my own internal engine—and my own way.

I want the same to happen for you, and that's why I wrote this book. I'm guiding you in the beginning here, but gradually you'll be able to take over the wheel and forge your own path to your goals. After all, the only path worth traveling on is your own. You will need courage and plenty of energy. Fortunately, you already have a store of unlimited fuel for your workout and your dreams inside you. The best way to access it? Training. The best place to use it? Everywhere.

Take the end of a sports match or a homework-filled night, for instance. Most guys have trouble sucking it up when pressure and fatigue hit. You, however, are different! You will train right, and train hard—then the exceptional path that only you are on will become that much easier to stay on. Going way beyond the easy ten reps in our workout will help you roar through the finish line and play better in the final period than in the first. Staying consistent with the workouts every week will push you to finish your schoolwork every night, participate in every class, and be admitted to the college of your choice.

Training has made all the difference for me. I try to get up earlier, work out harder, make more phone calls, meet more people, cut more deals than anybody else. Now, that's tough, but most important, I try to spend a lot of time with my family. As a result, a common question I hear from people is "Jake, where do you get all that energy?" The answer is many places, including an intense desire to make a good life for my family. But the number one source of energy is my workouts. There I push myself every time I train, and over time I have developed a huge pool of energy that's there for me anytime I need it. When I started my *Big Brother Jake* sitcom on the Family Channel, my unending supply of energy paid off because I could get up early enough to train, run my business, put in a full day at the set—then get up the next day and do it all again! Another energy source is my diet: I eat for energy as well as pleasure (more on that in Chapter 8).

Whether you want to be a rock musician or a rocket scientist, you will have to work at it for many hours to become a good one—and even more hours if you want to be a great one. Start training, and you'll develop the energy needed to put you over the top. It's in your hands—"it" being those Ferrari keys! Ready to start the engine?

MUSCLE MAKER: *Fueling the Tank Before Your Training Trip*

What's the most vital component of athletic performance, whether in your workout or during a game? Speed, power, and strength all rank up there, but they're all worthless without energy. That means you should go to your home gym or athletic field already pumped up! I always work out first thing in the morning because it is when I have the most energy. However, if you've spent the night cramming for an American History test, wait a day before you train again. It's crucial that you be well rested, especially if you work out several times a week. Your muscles need time to recover in between workouts.

If you plan to weight train or play a sport later in the day, eat a healthy meal about two to three hours before you lace your shoes up. Keep fat and protein on the low end, because they'll only slow you down. Instead, jack up the carbohydrate intake so you have that burst from the opening bell to the closing one. A sandwich on whole-wheat bread, pasta with vegetables, or a baked potato will all serve you well. Just make sure that in the hour before show time, you take in only fluids.

Be aware that your muscles, no matter how many carbs you've devoured that day, will still run dry if pushed too long and too hard. So if you've taken a long run or had a long sports practice, please don't try to lift weights afterward—your muscles will have nothing to go on! It's why you'll see many top-caliber athletes split their intense strength training and their cardiovascular work between morning and night or do them on different days; they can give full energy to both workouts, and their muscles will have recovered in the meantime. In addition, if you lose a lot of fluids during exercising because of your effort or the heat, use a sports drink to keep you hydrated and energetic!

▪ Take It on the Road ▪

I look my first steps to becoming a man down in my basement, because that's where I discovered weight training. Those weights helped me discover that inside my chubby exterior was a muscular dude waiting to shine! One thing was certain: before I started hitting those weights, nobody else was going to see anything special about me—from a good-looking girl to my English teacher to my basketball coach. I also wasn't headed anywhere near a Hollywood discovery story either! People liked me as out-of-shape Jake. Nobody thought I had to change, including my parents. It was up to me!

DREAM EXTREME: *From Frozen Tundra to Palm Trees*

Later in my teenage years, I was stuck somewhere else. Again, the only discovery to be made involving me had to come from me. I remember the moment as if it were yesterday—and I certainly remember the temperature! It was a bone-chilling day, with the windchill factor around twenty degrees below zero. I was wearing shorts and a mesh jersey with some pads underneath on a frozen lacrosse field in upstate New York. I was a freshman at Cortland State University playing for its lacrosse team, and we were scrimmaging Syracuse's team at its home field.

Let's put it this way: I wasn't having a blast, whether playing lacrosse that day or with anything else in school. I'd decided to go to Cortland State to please my parents. The problem was that it wasn't my goal; it was theirs. I knew that getting an education was the right thing to do, but for me that didn't mean it had to take place in college—especially in a place where my buttissimo was getting frozen off! I had friends and roommates who had come to college as part of their dream; guys and girls who wanted to be botanists and psychologists and journalists. My dreams, however, lay elsewhere.

My V-12 and I just didn't belong at Cortland State. I did try. I made the winter lacrosse team as a freshman; I studied as much as I could tolerate; I even landed the coolest job in town as a bouncer at the Shamrock—the only disco in town! The fact that my bouncer gig made me prouder than anything I did on the campus itself should have told me something, but I was too clueless to listen.

Only two weeks into my freshman year, I took cluelessness to another level. In an attempt to run for president of my dormitory, I set out to raise some "soft money" for my campaign by organizing "A Night in Las Vegas." In the common area, my buddies and I set up all the key Vegas ingredients: crap tables, blackjack, roulette. It was supposed to be low key, but word spread fast and we had about 450 people lined up to get in before we even dealt the first hand. The night ended before a dollar was made, however, when the dorm manager crashed the party and sent everybody home and almost sent me packing! I recall begging the guy, "Please don't tell my mom!" No, it wasn't my finest hour. The only place where my imagination and V-12 took me at Cortland State was trouble.

The great Jake-goes-to-college experiment ended as soon as I took my last spring semester final exam. I knew I wasn't coming back, because I decided I wasn't going to waste my parents' hard-earned money and my time anymore. My dream ever since I had first started lifting weights in my basement had been to be a bodybuilder, and suddenly I felt as though I had to go for it, right now. Cortland State was a perfect place for most of my peers and their dreams, but my dream was at home in a very different setting: the palm trees of L.A. Almost everybody thought I was doing fine at Cortland State and doubted L.A. would lead to anything. I knew better on both counts!

My message, however, isn't "Don't go to college." Quite the reverse: college is probably your most crucial pit stop before you take off on your career path, and I urge that you make it! I gave it a shot and realized it wasn't for me. That certainly doesn't mean it won't be for you!

Now it's your turn. Nobody knows your potential as well as you do, and we're going to pounce on it! We'll start by getting you into training, and then we'll put your dreams to work in motivating you to train harder and smarter. With every rep, you'll say to yourself "Princeton, Princeton, Princeton" or "great essay, great essay, great essay." You'll learn that these reps and your attempt to gain entry to a good college are connected because both are mostly dependent on effort. Later that day, when you sit down to write, you will be the determining force behind your application essay. Few people are willing to really focus and create a great one. You'll be different!

In your goals, the same rules apply: you do the work, you get by; you do more work, you get rewards. It's that simple. You have plenty of peers who do a "pretty good job" at studying for a test, defending against an opponent, or chatting up the new girl in school. You'll go further to get that A, to shut down the opposition's high scorer, or to be the first guy with the guts to ask that girl out.

As you can see, your V-12 is built for many places outside the gym. You'll start there, then go to many different arenas. You'll notice how training puts you in not only a good mood but an active mood, where you want to do additional things for yourself. That daily trip to Taco Bell with your friends won't seem so appealing now that your abs are starting to show. You'll go to the library to study up on your dream career rather than see *American Pie IX* for the fourth time!

▪ Use Your Own Compass ▪

Envy is a common emotion but a powerless one. While it is almost understandable in this celebrity-creating culture that we live in, if you examine any enviable person carefully, you'll find many flaws. Instead, place that person on the same level as you—even if he's Will Smith! Envy is always misplaced: respect is not. Respect him and his success, but, rather than trying to duplicate it, create your own success. Learn how he developed his talent and capitalized on it, then perfect your own method. By reading about my own trials and tribulations, you're finding out the ways to a better future—but you're not exactly like me. I can provide you with a map to muscles (see Chapter 5) and much more, but where you go with them is your decision!

An important tip: don't take the safe route that so many others travel on. If you're familiar with the traffic in L.A., that's only common sense! You see it every day, thousands upon thousands of people willing to sit in traffic rather than come up with a more inventive way to go from point A to point B. Take a risk and go on an alternative route: this will provide you with the bonus of showing you a different part of the city along the way. Risk takers get to their destinations, or goals, more quickly and experience much more in the process.

Taking risks usually means going against the tide. Risks shouldn't be taken randomly or thoughtlessly—don't play chicken with your nemesis or invite half your high school to your house when your parents are out of town. Instead, put plenty of thought into your actions before taking them. The very word "risk" means that there are serious potential consequences.

Maybe everybody studying a foreign language in your school thinks only Spanish or French is worthwhile, but you prefer Latin because it helps your understanding of words; or your friends think the unpopular girl in your class is pathetic, but you decide to ask her out because you can tell there's something special about her; or the entire basketball coaching staff wants you to play forward, but you insist on playing point guard because you know it'll make you a much better player.

What if your parents think studying Latin is a waste of time, your friends stop talking to you because you're dating the unpopular girl, or your coach makes you sit on the bench until you change your mind about being the point guard? Stick to your guns! A good risk can always be measured by the fact that you would have taken it no matter what the consequences. Sometimes it might take longer to pan out or for other people to adjust to your decision, but that comes with the territory. Leaving Cortland State was a risk that many people close to me thought was suspect at best, but it was one I never regretted—even though I struggled during my first couple of years in L.A.

A good risk is always worth taking because of its potential upside. You're automatically put into a more advanced league than those who don't take it. Your Latin studies may wind up helping you ace the verbal portion of the SAT, you might fall in love with the unpopular girl (and your friends may wind up thinking she's pretty cool, too), and you becoming point guard makes your team play better and your coach look like a genius! There aren't many short-cuts to success, but risk taking is definitely one of them.

Training supplies you with the guts to take your own path whenever the situation calls for it. You become more comfortable in your skin. Now you not only refuse to join your schoolmates who pick on the easy target—you know, the overweight or goofy guy—you befriend him. Maybe before you picked up those weights, you were the one who was picked on; now you want to keep it from happening to others.

I never liked being called "Typewriter" because of my stuttering or "Fat Boy" because I had a weight problem, but rather than fighting back with my fists, I used my weights. Soon I would never hear those words directed at me again, but I'd cringe—and still do to this day—when I heard them used about others. So whenever I got the chance, I did my best to put a stop to it, then and there. I'd love for you to do the same. That's what a leader does, and when you go your own way, that's what you will become (more on that in Chapter 7!).

REALITY CHECK: *Pick Your Own Jersey Number*

When you join a sports team, one of the hottest contests—even before you participate in your first practice—is who will snag the jersey numbers of your and your teammates' favorite professional players. It's even common among college athletes who want to be like their heroes, but all they end up doing is playing in their shadows. You'll notice again and again that all the greats—from Vince Carter's 15 to Derek Jeter's 2 to Brett Farve's 4—picked numbers that weren't highly sought after until they started wearing them! That's not a coincidence. I encourage you, too, to get your own number and create your own legacy!

Along the same lines, be a sports fan, but don't forget to participate yourself. If you habitually watch every televised football game every Sunday, that indicates to me that you're burying your own athletic interest in staring into a box rather than becoming a better athlete yourself. Have you ever noticed that most participants in sports trivia shows are out-of-shape lumps? That's also not a coincidence. Instead, watch a game only on a special occasion and let these great athletes inspire you to great feats of your own rather than simply motivating you to make another quick trip to the fridge and back before the commercials end!

▪ It's a New Day ▪

I'm disappointed whenever I wake up and can't remember any of my dreams. I think of those dreams that become my goals in much the same way. And there's no way my day won't be built on them. You, too, can base your day on your dreams, rather than allowing your dreams to be buried under an avalanche of day-to-day worries and concerns. Envision all the goals that you want to meet that day, even if the list runs a little long. You're not fine-tuning your mind and body just to loaf! You're ready to go full speed. As I tell myself, "If I can complete every set in my workout to the best of my ability, I should be able to easily complete the ten tasks I plan to tackle today."

Inevitably, you'll hit some potholes along the way, but I'm asking you to just power right through them. Whenever you take your V-12 farther along the road, you'll hit a few bumps, but you must keep your eyes on the road. Those who look back invariably hit another pothole. Keep looking ahead of you, and you'll forget all about the little troubles you have along the way. For example, maybe you missed the final shot of a game, the chance you had to speak to your favorite girl, or several biology pop quiz questions to which you knew the answer. Rather than getting hung up on those misses, anticipate the many future opportunities you'll have. Here's the next part of the poem "Don't Quit":

DON'T QUIT POEM: *Stay on That Road!*

Life is queer with its twists and turns,
As every one of us sometimes learns,
And many a failure turns about
When he might have won had he stuck it out;
Don't give up though the pace seems slow—
You may succeed with another blow.

To stay on course, instill some good habits into yourself. Number one is time management. I try never to squander my time on anything not worthwhile. As a result, you will never see me camped out in front of the television for the evening, clicking away at espn.go.com for an hour, or sleeping in. As mentioned earlier, the amount of muscle energy you have is finite, but so is your energy for your daily tasks. Spending your alert hours on such activities wastes time that you could turn toward much more productive ones.

Break down your week and see if you can spot the time wasters: the hour phone call that could have lasted ten minutes; watching an entire game versus just the fourth quarter; or goofing around with your friends after school for two hours instead of twenty minutes. I'm not recommending that you cut out all these parts of your life but that you limit the time spent on things that have nothing to do with your goals.

Good habits and bad habits cannot coexist peacefully, so the more good habits you have, the better the chance that your bad habits will go away. For example, maybe you always feel that you're behind from the moment you wake up. So get an early start on the day! Maybe you won't join me at 5 A.M., but start by getting up an hour earlier than your normal time (and going to bed earlier, too). You'll be surprised at how much more you get done.

Maybe you're notoriously late for everything. Set your watch twenty minutes early, then you will never be late. Perhaps you have trouble getting in a workout. Then make the early morning your time to train. I always train in the morning, because I'm more rested and then my workout's out of my way for the rest of the day. Best of all, it energizes me for the *entire* day!

POWER HABIT: *The Power List*

Interested to know what my biggest secret of a successful day is apart from training? It's my things-to-do list—a true fundamental of mental fitness. Each night, take out a notepad and plan out how your next day will go. This list will help you operate at peak efficiency, partly because you won't waste energy trying to remember what needs to be done and when.

What I like most about the Power List is that it gives you direction and purpose. You're forced to think about what will make for a successful day, which means you should include your dreams and goals on the list. You won't be able to fit all of them in, but conceiving a few things you can do to further a dream or get closer to a goal will make all the difference in the long run. This practice ensures that your day won't be dominated by tasks and events unrelated to your goals. Maybe you have a task you're not looking forward to, such as vacuuming the house, but also on your list is your plan to learn a new computer program that relates to your desire to become a computer engineer one day.

Meanwhile, many of the tasks on the list should be relatively easy to accomplish, so when you look back on your day, you're guaranteed to have some wins. For example, eating a healthy breakfast and studying solidly during your free period aren't gargantuan tasks, but they still belong on the list!

I always begin my list with old business that I didn't finish that day, loose ends I want to tie up first thing the following day. Next I make my list in order of importance, with the big activities at the top of it. I always leave room for notes, which then makes my notebook a useful reference tool for whenever I need to refer to it. Save each day's lists, then look back on them weeks or months later whenever you want evidence of your progress!

The next day, stick to your list by referring to it periodically. Cross out each task as you finish it, which frees your mind to move on to the next item. By the end of the day, when you're about to create another list, put today behind and focus on tomorrow.

By the time your active day is done and your homework finished, you're probably more than ready to hit the sack. However, there are a couple of things left. First is an evening pep talk, in which you ask yourself two key questions: What did I accomplish today? How can I build on what I learned today? These accomplishments don't need to be grand. Maybe you finally spoke up in class or you said "Hi" to your dream girl. Those are achievements that will lead you closer to your goals. The lessons of your day might include listening more carefully to your coach in practice, resulting in him taking more notice of your good playing, or recognizing that your best friend had fun being in the school play, causing you to consider trying out next time around. These aren't huge lessons, but they will add up to make you a happier, more successful person.

Second, start off on the right foot the next day by getting yourself geared up the night before. I'm talking about not only getting pumped up mentally about a promising day, but getting set up physically as well. Plan what you're going to have for breakfast by making sure it's in the kitchen. Determine your clothes for the day by checking the weather forecast. Pack your backpack with your books and gym/sports practice clothes, then put your wallet and key on top of them. If you work out at home, put your workout clothes in a pile nearby so they're the first thing you put on in the morning. Stick your things-to-do list right beside your bed so it's the first thing you see in the morning.

Armed with these habits, you'll start every day on the right foot and in the right frame of mind. Finally, you will have time to tackle your work and your dreams! Are you getting pumped up? I hope so, because the Muscle Quotient tests are next. Get ready!

THE MQ TESTS

four

Still having trouble with that mirror test? Not sure what you need to work on? Good. That's why I created the MQ (Muscle Quotient) tests. You've heard of the IQ test, which measures intelligence; well, the MQ tests measure your muscles. However, you won't be breaking out the tape measure, because MQ has nothing to do with muscle size.

Instead, MQ sets a new fitness standard that evaluates exactly how well your muscles function. Through these eight tests, you will determine your present level of strength, endurance, power, aerobic capacity, balance, coordination, and flexibility—the whole enchilada. Unlike tests in school, though, the MQ tests are a lot more fun and can be taken completely on your own. Neither a PE teacher nor a coach will stand over you; and twenty other classmates or teammates won't be watching. It's just you—ready to challenge yourself?

After completing each test, you'll plug your result into a simple formula that will spit out a score. Each test includes four different levels and enables you to see how you stack up against your teenage peers for each category. Maybe you kick butt on the one-mile run but can't pull off many pull-ups. Maybe you come up short on the vertical leap, but can do stomach curl-ups until the sun goes down. Either way, there's no more guesswork about what your strengths and weaknesses are. After you're finished with all the tests, tabulate your total to find out which camp you're in.

Even if your ego gets bruised more than boosted with these tests, taking them is an important step. You're now acknowledging what your physical weaknesses are, not just how you look in the mirror. If you truly want to *look, feel, and be powerful,* it's time to find out what you need to work on. Remember: the MQ tests are different from any other test, for they represent only the beginning, not the end, of preparing yourself to get into the best shape possible! People say your IQ score can never be improved, but MQ is a different story. The results are never final!

DREAM EXTREME: *Get to Your Goals!*

Don't worry if you come up short in many of the tests or your total score puts you in the camp where everybody sleeps in. You have to evaluate to excel! MQ tells you where you're at, not where you're going. You're ready to go far, so let's set some goals! It takes you nine minutes to run a mile? Try to knock it down to eight. Have trouble cranking out a dozen push-ups? Aim for twenty. Even if you scored pretty well in some of these tests, set a goal for a better score. Ultimately, I want you to write down a goal for every single test.

Next I'll help you determine how to reach those goals. One way is to take these tests again and again, since some of them are a workout in themselves! However, to really do better on any test, you need to prepare. In the next chapter, I give you the map to muscle and more. Follow all the directions week after week, and your muscles will get stronger and faster while you go longer and harder than ever before. Retake the MQ tests a month from now, and you'll see your score jump! Keep up the exercises, and every month your score will go up another notch.

Meanwhile, you will also do better at the other tests that come your way—your first visit to a college campus, your first practice with the soccer team, your first day of school after summer break—especially if you set goals in those areas as well. You improved your mile time by two minutes? Imagine what you can do with your SAT score. You can now perform seventeen toe touches in thirty seconds? Think how much better your goalie skills will be. Improve in all areas over the summer, and your classmates will be guaranteed to notice next fall!

To bring more fun into the MQ journey, recruit a buddy to join you. It'll make it even easier to score, plus the competition will probably increase both your scores!

Since some tests are tougher than others, follow the order suggested. Block out an hour and go to work. MQ may make you pretty sore, however, so wait at least one day before you start the Get Strong! workout. To record your results accurately, use a pencil, notepad, calculator, and stopwatch.

Let the games begin!

MQ TEST 1: Toe Touches

MQ kicks off with a test that will get your muscles warmed up, and it's not as easy as it looks. Intended to measure your coordination as well as your hand and foot speed, you actually train your brain to move your muscles more quickly. You may feel very uncoordinated during your first go-through, but your coordination will improve if you do this drill frequently. In any sport where possession of the ball and doing something special with it is important—from football to juggling!—you'll be better off with this skill.

TEST YOURSELF: Stand up with your knees slightly bent and torso upright. Raise your left leg, bring your left foot out in front of you, and touch your toe with your right hand as quickly as you can; then touch your right foot with your left hand in the same way. Next, touch your left foot behind your body with your right hand, then your right foot with your left hand behind your body. Repeat as fast as you can over the course of thirty seconds.

HOW TO SCORE: Multiply the number of touches completed (only a total circuit counts) by 5.

YOUR RESULTS:

NUMBER COMPLETED	RATING	SCORE
0–8	Wake-up call!	0–40
9–12	Showing some signs!	45–60
13–16	Your V-12 is humming!	65–80
17+	BMOC material!	85+

MQ TEST 2: One-Leg Stand

Having good balance often means the difference between smoothly finishing a move in whatever sport you play and landing hard on your buttissimo! Similar to toe touches in that you're training your brain to recognize the difference between balance and not, it's a vital skill because in most sports you're frequently caught off balance. If you can recover quickly, however, your chances of success go up. Test yourself today, then start working on this one-legged business several times a week—while you're on the phone, brushing your teeth, or practicing a speech!—and make sure you practice on both legs!

TEST YOURSELF: Using bare feet (shoes make it easier), stand straight up and bend one knee to lift your foot a few inches off the ground behind you. Look straight ahead with your hands on your hips, then start the timer and close your eyes. Balance on your one straight leg for as long as you can.

HOW TO SCORE: See what category your time falls into. For example, 42 seconds and 1 minute 29 seconds both count the same, 72 points.

YOUR RESULTS:

TIME	RATING	SCORE
0–20 seconds	Wake-up call!	10
21–40 seconds	Showing some signs!	45
41 seconds–1 minute 30 seconds	Your V-12 is humming!	72
1 minute 31 seconds and up	BMOC material!	100

MQ TEST 3: Vertical Leap

If you play ball, any kind of ball, you already know how invaluable the ability to get off the ground is. Unfortunately, many of us think we either can or can't jump, so few people work on it. However, it's like any other skill: it can be learned. In the next chapter, I will give you a couple of drills that will have you climbing the wall!

TEST YOURSELF: Cover the fingertips of your dominant hand with chalk (or any other substance that will wash off, such as dirt). Stand one foot away from a wall, facing it and with your feet, hips, and shoulders parallel to it. Reach up as high as you can on your tiptoes and touch the wall. Next, quickly bend your hips and knees into a half-squatting position, then explode vertically upward and mark a spot on the wall at the apex of your jump with your fingertips. Measure the difference.

HOW TO SCORE: Multiply the number of inches jumped by 2.5.

YOUR RESULTS:

INCHES	RATING	SCORE
0–17	Wake-up call!	0–42.5
17.1–21	Showing some signs!	42.8–52.5
21.1–27	Your V-12 is humming!	52.8–67.5
27.1+	BMOC material!	67.8+

MQ TEST 4: Curl-up

Flat, defined abs can be your vanity plates, but with the abdominal muscles there's much more than meets the eye. Your "core" also holds much of your power and control. In any sport, from skateboarding to wrestling, a strong core makes you a much more competitive athlete and less prone to injury. Meanwhile, when you sit on your duff for hours on end studying, a good set of abs helps your back from getting stiff! I take my abs so seriously that I make sure they're always the first muscle group I train whenever I work out.

TEST YOURSELF: Lie down on a padded surface with your knees slightly bent at a 140-degree angle, feet flat on the floor, legs slightly apart. Place your arms straight and parallel to your trunk with your palms face down on the mat. Begin with your head resting on the mat, then curl your trunk up until you feel your upper abs contract and your fingers are pushed a few inches forward. Then curl back down until your head touches the mat. Your heels remain on the mat. Keep your head still and aligned with your trunk. Follow a cadence of one curl-up every 3 seconds. Continue without pausing until you can no longer do any more or have completed 75 reps.

HOW TO SCORE: Multiply the number of 3-second reps completed by 1.35.

YOUR RESULTS:

NUMBER COMPLETED	RATING	SCORE
0–15	Wake-up call!	0–20.3
16–34	Showing some signs!	21.6–45.9
35–59	Your V-12 is humming!	47.3–79.7
60+	BMOC material!	81+

MQ TEST 5: Pull-ups

Just as "pulling your own weight" one day in the future will be a man-sized test, so is this one with the pull-up bar. If you're well set up with muscle and little fat, you'll probably be able to rip off a number of them. But if you are carrying any extra flab, even if it's accompanied by plenty of muscle, you'll be punished because you have to pull it into the air. In addition, unless you're already lifting weights and/or make a habit of hanging from trees, your back muscles probably haven't seen a lot of action. As a result, don't get down on yourself if you can't do even a single one. Use the exercises in the next chapter to change that in a hurry!

TEST YOURSELF: You need to own a pull-up apparatus for this test, and any sporting goods shop will carry one. (You'll also need it—along with a few other items detailed in the next chapter—for the upcoming Get Strong! workout.) Use a horizontal bar at a height that allows you to hang with your arms fully extended and feet clear of the floor. Take an overhand, shoulder-width grip on the bar. Pull your shoulder blades down and keep them there throughout the exercise. Use your arms and back to pull your body up as your elbows go out until your chin is above the bar, then lower to the start position. Don't swing your body or kick your legs. Do as many as you can; there is no time limit.

HOW TO SCORE: Multiply the number of pull-ups completed by 4.

YOUR RESULTS:

NUMBER COMPLETED	RATING	SCORE
0–4	Wake-up call!	0–16
5–9	Showing some signs!	20–36
10–19	Your V-12 is humming!	40–76
20+	BMOC material!	80+

MQ TEST 6: Push-ups

If you want to know how strong you are for your size, this is *the* test. There's no better way to measure the explosive power and endurance strength of your upper body. A bench press is a breeze by comparison, because a push-up forces so many muscles to work—naturally, the chest, shoulders, and triceps take their fair share of the load, but the muscles of your forearms, wrists, stomach, lower back, and even legs help keep you in the air as well. In fact, whenever I'm someplace where I don't have any access to equipment and need an upper-body pump, this is always my first go-to exercise.

TEST YOURSELF: Assume a prone position on the mat with hands placed under your shoulders, fingers stretched out, legs straight and slightly apart, and toes tucked under. Push off the mat with your arms until they're straight, while keeping your legs and back straight. Lower your body until your elbows bend to 90 degrees and your upper arms are parallel to the floor. Push back to the start position. Do as many as you can in one minute; you may tire before the time is up, so pace yourself.

HOW TO SCORE: Multiply the number of push-ups completed by 1.7.

YOUR RESULTS:

NUMBER OF PUSH-UPS	RATING	SCORE
0–12	Wake-up call!	0–20.4
13–24	Showing some signs!	22.1–40.8
25–45	Your V-12 is humming!	42.5–76.5
46+	BMOC material!	78.2+

MQ TEST 7: One-Mile Run

If you've had a long layoff or think that running shoes are only a style choice, this might be the test you dread the most. The one-mile run is all about aerobic capacity, and that's at its best only if you've built it up over time. With so many sports matches and races coming down to the final stretches, endurance really is the ultimate weapon. No matter what level you're at, set a goal to go faster to improve your sporting success. See the next chapter for more information on how to develop aerobic power.

TEST YOURSELF: Choose a flat running course one mile long. If you use a 400-meter track, go four laps plus 10 yards. You may also use a treadmill on a flat level. Start your timer. Remember, this is a lot longer than down to the 7-Eleven and back, so pace yourself. Wait to come on strong at the end.

HOW TO SCORE: Multiply your total seconds by 0.3, then subtract that total from 175.

YOUR RESULTS:

TIME (MIN:SEC)	RATING	SCORE
9:00+	Wake-up call!	0–13
8:59–6:15	Showing some signs!	13.3–62.5
6:14–5:01	Your V-12 is humming!	62.8–84.7
5:00 and below	You're BMOC material!	85+

MQ TEST 8: Sit and Stretch

The lower back goes through a lot of twists and turns in your daily sporting activities, and unless it's flexible, it may decide to quit on you. To keep both it and you in the game, start stretching your hamstrings and lower back area several times a week. Here's a test to see where you're at right now.

TEST YOURSELF: Sit flat on the ground with your legs stretched out in front of you. Place your hands on top of your knees and keep your spine erect. Bending from your hips (not your back!) and flexing your thigh muscles (makes it easier to stretch your hamstrings), move your hands forward along the top of your straight legs. Go slowly until you feel a stretch and hold. Remember, never stretch to the point of pain.

HOW TO SCORE: Check to see how far your fingertips reached and compare to chart below.

YOUR RESULTS:

REACH DISTANCE	RATING	SCORE
Knee to midshin	Wake-up call!	10
Lower shin	Showing some signs!	45
Ankle area	Your V-12 is humming!	72
Foot or beyond	You're BMOC material!	100

YOUR MQ TOTAL

TOTAL POINTS	SCORE
0–199	Wake-up call!: You now know all the areas where you need to get better. Let's go for it!
200–399	Showing some signs!: Work on your weaknesses, and you'll be jumping up a spot soon.
400–599	Your V-12 is humming!: Great performance! Continue to crank away, and even more improvement will take place.
600–799	BMOC material!: You're among the elite. Keep up the good work, and start carrying your prowess over to different kinds of successes.

THE MAP TO MUSCLES
AND MANHOOD

The MQ tests showed you where you are on the map, and you probably have a good idea where you want to go—your very own MGM Studio! You know, muscles, girls, and manhood! To drive your powerful engine through those formidable gates onto that star-studded lot, however, takes a lot of guts and know-how. I can supply you with the know-how; the guts are up to you.

The map begins and ends with my workout, which I humbly(!) consider the greatest one out there. It will be your source for everything—not just the physical stuff like muscles, strength, endurance, and speed, but also for gaining confidence, energy, a clear mind, inspiration, and good looks! Refer to this map frequently, and be faithful to it. The rewards will be greater than you can possibly imagine.

When I first started training down in my basement, it hit me: this was an activity I could do completely on my own and never get bored. If I ever did, I simply challenged myself more or changed the exercises. I wasn't the sort of teenage guy who closed the door and curled up with a book, so instead I closed the door and curled a barbell. It became my private space that I looked forward to every day and where I grew both physically and mentally.

While I enjoyed hanging out with my buddies as much as before, I was no longer dependent on them for the everyday entertainment provided by playing basketball or going cruising. Now I had my own thing, and it made me feel better than beating my buddy six times in a row in a game of H-O-R-S-E or talking with a carful of beautiful girls. My training was better, because it worked for me every time.

In *your* basement, *your* room, *your* gym, wherever you train, that's where it's going to happen for you. That's the place where you'll gain muscle and confidence, and start on your way toward your goals.

YOUR TRAINING TOOLS

I'd love to tell you that a chair and padded floor are enough to train with, but that would ultimately sell your muscles short. Instead, spend (or kindly ask your parents to help) a couple hundred bucks or less for your very own home gym. Go to your nearest sporting goods shop, check out a used–sporting goods store, or look on the Web.

If buying this equipment means spending two and a half weeks' worth of lawn-mowing money, remember: this is an investment in your future. And unlike the volatile stock market, this one's a sure winner! These are the things you'll need:

1. Weight bench, with incline. Leg curl and leg extension apparatuses are helpful but not essential.

2. Straight bar.

3. Two dumbbell bars.

4. At least 150 pounds of weights. You probably won't use them all now, but you will soon! These weights should fit on both the straight bar and dumb-bell bars.

5. Pull-up bar. Get one to fit in a door frame or a heavier-duty apparatus to put up in the garage.

6. Dynamic tension bands. Several brands exist. They will be used for leg curls, unless you already have the apparatus as part of your bench.

▪ The Most Challenging Hour of Your Life ▪

Your muscles are about to see more action than they've ever seen—in a workout that lasts only one hour. What's the secret? Putting no limits on yourself. Most workouts have you spending more than half the time resting, but here every minute is accounted for. The do-one-set-then-take-a-long-break concept is thrown out the window. In its place are faster-paced workouts that bring out as much muscle potential as possible.

What are the advantages? Where do I start? First, your month is broken down into four different workouts, so your muscles never get a chance to coast. You challenge them differently each week rather than doing the same routine again and again. As a result, you hit every muscle fiber of each body part in every conceivable way, guaranteeing maximum muscle growth.

Second, the total volume of sets and reps adds up to phenomenal endurance strength, which is much more useful in sports and the everyday world than brute strength. Unless you're hoping to be a power lifter or shot putter, strength over time and distance is what counts. Look at "power" sports such as football or even sumo wrestling: while these athletes need a burst of strength initially, they then have to carry on with that strength another ten seconds or much longer on a football field or wrestling mat—even if they weigh more than three hundred pounds! In other sports, quickness (which I'll help you with as well) seems to reign superior, but it's guys who can play hard all day long who succeed, whether in basketball, soccer, tennis, surfing, or any other sport.

Third, you get a great cardiovascular benefit, with your heart rate jumping up as you start burning through the calories. As a result, if you have any extra flab, this workout will take care of it on top of the muscle making.

Fourth, you receive the same benefits (and then some) in half the time as with the routines written up in the muscle magazines, leaving you plenty of time for your other activities and goals that day. Remember: fitness is the means to achieve other good things, not the be-all and end-all (that's for the chuckleheads!).

This workout is not a piece of cake. If it were, everybody would be in great shape! So you will be tested mentally. You will be tempted to give in to the first signs of fatigue with each set, to finish off a muscle group later, to put off the workout to another day. However, you won't submit, because you have accepted the challenge! You want to see not only how much you can lift but also how long you can lift it! You're ready to work a muscle until it has nothing left! You're committed to training with me three to four times a week and you will not miss a single workout!

TIPS FOR TRAINING SUCCESS

Teenage life is hectic, with a heavy schedule of school, sports, and extracurricular activities, plus the obligations of family life. Here are some ways to overcome the many competing distractions and stay on your training track.

1. Get the workout in. That means, do whatever you can to stay on schedule. Designate an hour in your day when you can train; maybe it's after school or during a midevening homework break. Try always to make it at the same time; then it will become a habit. Link your muscles with that training day, and keep them there. Too much to do after school one day? Work out in the morning. Have only twenty minutes to spare? Train as hard as you can for those twenty minutes. All that being said, if you still miss your workout, don't beat yourself up about it—your gains won't vanish overnight! Instead, come up with a time the next day when you can make it up, then push your whole schedule back a day that week. Next week you'll be back in the saddle.

2. Find the perfect spot. Smack-dab in front of the TV won't work too well, and neither will a room where disaster awaits every lunge and curl— whoops, there goes Mom's favorite vase! Instead, locate a space where you can set up shop, so each time you work out you don't have to pull everything out from under the bed. Have it ready to go, then you can get right down to business! The garage and basement are usually great places, or your room if it's big enough.

3. Bare bones is better. The weight belt, weight gloves, wrist straps, knee wraps—they aren't needed. The weight belt is supposed to protect your lower back but instead just weakens your stomach muscles. With the other devices, you're able to lift more weight; however, building strength around the joints by not using them is much more beneficial than the ability to overload a muscle group with them. If you can't handle a weight with sweaty hands or wobbly knees, it's too heavy!

4. Sometimes help is needed. Some days the blood isn't pumping as you want it to and couch crashing sounds a lot more appealing. Get some music that puts you back in the training mood fast. Whether it's hip-hop or hard rock, put on whatever works to get you motivated again. A training partner, if

chosen well, can also boost your training level. Don't try to take on a "project" (a less advanced workout partner) until you have these workouts down pat. Instead, choose somebody who's at your level or, even better, above—a friend or family member, for example—and who's as pumped up about training as you are. I train with a partner whenever I can, to increase the challenge and make it more fun.

▪ The DQ Zone ▪

From the MQ tests to the DQ Zone. No, it's not a trip to Dairy Queen to reward yourself! DQ stands for "Don't Quit," words that I've lived by since I was given that poem in eighth grade. The DQ Zone is the mental space I want you to enter every time you train. Then nothing else will throw you off your game for the rest of the day.

If you give your workout everything you have from the first exercise and stay there, you're in the DQ Zone. At every training session, potential excuses and surrender will be defeated by your consistency and intensity. You'll be amazed at how far your body can take you by your simply raising the level each and every time you train. I still do it, and you don't want to even hear the insane numbers I can throw at you. Well, here are two: how do 1,000 reps in fourteen minutes sound? I did that the other day, but don't try that workout at home!

To belong in this zone, you've got to be jacked up. Use whatever you can to motivate you. Want to look good in front of others? There's nothing wrong with that. Don't think you have the genes to get huge or be fast? Prove yourself wrong—you just haven't worked hard enough! Getting ready for beach or soccer season? Are you desperate to beat your brother in one-on-one? Get focused and go to work!

If you train with a partner or at a gym, be aware that the DQ Zone doesn't mean a lot of chatter. Quite the reverse; you're in what I term "silent training camp." Back when I trained Harrison Ford, we had much fun because he was such a superintense, no-nonsense type of guy. I'd get him doing push-ups while counting them off, then I'd slowly pick up the pace until he'd shoot me one of his famous glares. I'd read it to mean "Hey, pal, I can count, too." That's how we came up with the idea of a silent training camp. Leave the idle talk for later, and stay inside your mind.

TRAINING TRIP-UPS: *Gain Without the Pain*

Whoever said "no pain, no gain" has a lot to answer for! With injuries more common than ever among athletes and weight lifters, be mindful of these training rules:

1. Start small no matter how big you want to become. The important thing is intensity, not poundage, which will come naturally. As it is, you'll experience some muscle soreness and stiffness with this routine; go too heavy, however, and suddenly you'll have an unwanted guest at your party: injury!

2. Steer clear of power-lifting moves. Power lifting—quick, explosive Olympic-style moves like the dead lift and clean and jerk—is still used by many athletes, but it's a joint wrecker and won't do anything more for you or your sport than my routine. In fact, power lifting is really as sport-specific as swinging a golf club is for golfers. In other words, leave power lifting to power lifters.

3. Watch for signs of overtraining. You should never begin a workout for any muscle that is still sore. (If any of your other muscles that you're not going to train that day is sore, however, that's okay.) Excessive fatigue after a workout or at random times during the day is also an indication that you're overdoing it. Lack of sleep can be a big contributor to overtraining, so get your eight hours!

4. Listen to your joints. I've eliminated all the exercises that sometimes cause joint problems, but that doesn't mean that one of these exercises won't still trigger some joint pain. Everybody is designed differently, so naturally some exercises don't work for certain types of body frames. For example, I have a buddy who is six feet, four inches tall who uses only dumbbells because straight bars—and especially machines in the gym—don't work for his long arms. If you ever feel persistent pain in your shoulder, elbow, wrist, or knee, for instance, try substituting a different exercise and often the pain will disappear. Then put that problematic exercise on the "not for me" list.

▪ Brain Train ▪

We're almost to the workout, I promise! Before you start to expand your muscles, however, you need to expand your mind. Going through an entire workout with thoughts no more advanced than "my chest, my chest, my chest" or "one more rep" is an opportunity wasted! Instead of being a brain drain, a good workout fills your brain with power!

I noticed this right away when I began training. I looked in the mirror and said, "If I can lift these weights ten times, I can do whatever I want." And I did those reps. Then I challenged myself to do fifteen, and so on. After a while, all the teenage stuff I was dealing with—nervousness, aggression, not speaking in class, being embarrassed about how I looked—was taken out on that iron.

Start to incorporate your goals into the workout by reciting each one on every lift. Visualize that each lift takes you a step closer to that goal—whether within your workout, that week in school, or down the road. Your muscles will then grow in tandem with your confidence, as you realize that nothing that day will be as tough as the workout you have just given your body and mind. Suddenly, you will be better equipped to deal with anything that comes your way, from a golden opportunity to a rotten egg.

Ask yourself: How much muscle do you want? How badly do you want to go to a top college? How much do you want to ask out that girl in history class? Tell yourself that five more reps gives you five more pounds of muscle, five application letters, five chances to make a great impression on her. After every workout, not only will those dreams be more real in your mind, but you will be readier to tackle the work that's needed to make them happen.

After your tough workout, it will be a relief to sit down and study. Your body will welcome the chance to take a comfortable seat and begin reading and writing. Your mind will be free of clutter and ready to concentrate.

THE GET STRONG! WORKOUT

Finally, here it is, what you've been waiting for: the workout. The ultimate goal of this workout plan is to maximize your strength and muscle gains. Split into four separate training weeks—each emphasizing a different form of strength conditioning—it will give you and your muscles the best chance to do exactly that.

To take advantage of that chance, however, you will have to make an intense effort—for no matter how great this program is, the key ingredient in maximizing your strength and muscle is what you put into it. That means that when you feel as though you've done the last rep you can, do another four! Believe me, your muscles will be capable if you let *your mind* push them. Practice this method for every set, and you will be floored at how fast your muscles and strength increase.

Consequently, when you see only two exercises and three sets of each for your chest, I expect you to go full-tilt boogie on each of those sets to the point that doing any more would be pointless! Such a high-intensity approach, in fact, makes full use of your energy *and* muscle potential—while also delivering an incredibly time-efficient workout.

Hitting each muscle group twice a week, meanwhile, ensures the best athletic conditioning. You'll not only get the muscle size you want but also develop durable and active muscles that will be more usable than ever. This includes training muscles that normally don't get any attention in regular weight-lifting routines. So beyond the chest and the biceps exercises, I also give you moves for other areas of your body that need to be strong for you to be at your best and avoid injury. They include the rotator cuff—which is susceptible to tears in any sport, especially those involving throwing, unless it's trained—and the lower back.

Do you know why feeling sore after a great workout feels good? It's because you did something good for yourself that you now carry around with you. It's a reminder of a success out of which many more will spring. It's going to be a great month. Let's go!

THE PERFECT REP WITH THE PERFECT WEIGHT

These two fundamental parts of lifting are often misunderstood. Learn how to lift exactly right, and you will never shortchange your muscles!

1. Observe form over content: Follow the exercise descriptions and pictures carefully to get maximum muscle benefit while preventing injury.

2. A repetition is the number of successful contractions performed during each exercise. A set is the total number of repetitions you perform in an exercise, from start to finish, before resting.

3. Slow down: Lifting a weight too quickly doesn't work your muscles thoroughly for three reasons: (A) It means you're probably using too light a weight. (B) Fewer muscle fibers are involved. (C) It creates momentum, which in turn takes the strain off and the benefit away from your muscle. The best tempo is about two seconds up and four seconds down.

4. Let yourself breathe: Good breathing helps your lifting power. Inhale on the preparation phase of the rep, then exhale completely on the effort phase.

5. Feel the muscle: For whatever muscle you're targeting, concentrate on flexing the muscle through the entire movement in order to get more development.

6. Pause: In the position of full muscle contraction, pause briefly.

7. Choose your weight wisely: The ideal weight for you is when you're barely able to make it into the prescribed rep range. Fall short? Lower the weight. Get there without trouble? Up it. For some exercises, weight increases and decreases may be as little as 2.5 pounds per side.

▪ The Preseason: You Started with the MQ Tests, Now Go On to the SQ Test! ▪

Before you jump into Week 1 of the program, a preseason period will help you prepare to pump! First, take the MQ tests in Chapter 4 to see where your muscles are at. Second, hit the weights to make them better! But don't hit them too hard if you've never lifted before. Instead, do just one set of the exercises listed below. Do between 12 and 15 reps after a warm-up set. Do all the exercises in one session, then wait three days before repeating the same workout. So if you worked out on Monday, go again on Thursday.

Three days later, take the SQ test. The "strength quotient" test represents exactly what your strength levels are right now for each muscle. As valuable as the MQ tests, it tells you where you're strong and where you're not. Plan on upping your poundage on every exercise by the time you take it at the beginning of every month, and watch your SQ and MQ scores skyrocket!

If you have worked out before, take the SQ test right out of the gate. Then wait at least four days before beginning Week 1.

To do the SQ test, take the following percentage of your body weight for each exercise, then complete as many full reps as possible. You will need a calculator! Do a very thorough warm-up set, going about twenty reps with a relatively light weight. See the exercise descriptions later in the chapter to make sure you do each test correctly. (All exercises listed below involve a straight bar, unless otherwise noted.)

1. Chest: Flat Bench Press with 50 percent of your total weight (page 71)
2. Shoulders: Standing Military Press with 30 percent (page 87)
3. Triceps: Lying Dumbbell French Press with 20 percent (page 88)
4. Back: Bent-Over Row with 35 percent (page 90)
5. Biceps: Standing Barbell Curl with 20 percent (page 78)
6. Quadriceps: Squat with 50 percent (page 75)
7. Hamstrings: Leg Curl (with dynamic band or 25 percent with apparatus) (page 76)
8. Calves: One-Legged Calf Raise with no weight (page 77)

After you finish each exercise, write down how many reps you did. At the end, total them. First, try to do more than ten reps of each exercise, then twenty, thirty, and on! Later, compare all these numbers each time you take the SQ test. Be prepared to see big changes!

Enough talk, let's get busy!

GO FASTER, GO LONGER, GO HIGHER

Hitting the weights hard four times a week will go a long way toward creating muscle and athletic power, but if you want to go further—to the "V-12" and "BMOC" levels of the MQ tests—you need to build a serious cardiovascular component into your routine. No matter what sport you play, there are some common abilities that translate into athletic success: running faster and longer, jumping higher and more explosively, as well as moving from side to side and back and forth more quickly and powerfully. Even if you're a natural athlete, these abilities don't develop unless you work on them week after week.

Instead of handing you a program, though, I want you to design your own with the following concepts. Maybe you prefer to bike, row, or climb stairs rather than run. Maybe you're interested only in endurance running and care little about how high you can jump. I urge you to pick the concepts that appeal to you and make them your own. If all four sound worth working hard for, decrease the initial recommendations by half. Overall, begin slowly the first couple of weeks, then go up a level once your body adjusts and start pushing it!

· *Run all day long without even breathing hard.* The old-school method of improving your aerobic capacity is simply to run long distances several days a week. But this puts you at a risk for overuse injuries such as shin splints and knee problems, plus possibly getting bored to death. A better way is to continue to run three to four days a week, for example, but to go for different distances at different speeds. One week, go 4 miles on Sunday, 1.5 on Tuesday, 2.5 on Thursday, then finish on Friday with 0.5. For the shorter-distance days, go harder. As time passes, slowly add to each day's distance if you choose.

· *Become flat-out fast.* Running uphill adds resistance to your body and forces more fast-twitch fibers (the parts of your muscle that give you the "burst") to come alive. Your ability to explode off the starting line plus keep up your speed for short distances will be greatly enhanced. Begin on a slight incline and sprint up about 15 yards at 80 percent effort. Walk back, then repeat, four times in all. The last one should be an all-out effort. Do twice a week. Choose a hill with a steeper incline, increase the length of sprint, or the numbers of reps each week.

· *Get game speed and game recovery.* Ever notice that no matter how hard you practice, a game is still tougher? That's because a game is always faster, in both the speed of the players and the shortness of the rest intervals. (It also has something to do with all those girls in the bleachers.) If you order up a "sprint and float" for yourself, however, game day will be a cinch. Use a treadmill or some other soft surface (grass or a cushioned track, for example) to sprint vigorously for a set period or distance, then throttle down into "float" mode for an equal, longer, or shorter period or distance, then repeat any number of times. The key is to stay relaxed and get the motion down. Eventually, your sprint will become your float! A ten-minute session of thirty-second sprints and floats three times a week is a good place to start. Then gradually ratchet up the amount of time spent sprinting each week.

· *Climb the air.* In any ball-oriented sport, the guy who jumps higher is usually the one who gets the props—shagging a fly ball over the wall, dunking in traffic, heading a ball toward the goal. To help your "hops," do these two drills twice a week for three sets. On grass or a cushioned wood floor, stand relaxed and upright with your feet about shoulder width apart. (1) Towel Jump. Face a rolled-up towel on the ground and jump over it quickly, then jump backward over it. Maintain good body control and athletic posture throughout. Continue for twenty total touches. Limit your time on the ground as much as possible. (2) Jump Squat. Clasp your hands behind your head. Squat downward to a half-squat position, then explode upward as high as possible, extending your hips, knees, and ankles to their maximum length as quickly as you can. For the first couple of weeks, freeze the landing, check your posture, then repeat. Progress to multiple reps without rest in between. Do 4 to 8 reps.

STRETCHING: TRAIN AND RECOVER AT YOUR BEST

Stretching is the most overlooked part of training. However, it's essential: it helps prevent injury, betters your lifting and sports performance, plus improves your posture. A great time to stretch is right after you've taken your postworkout shower, because your muscles are more limber and just begging to be stretched! Plus that long towel will come in handy for a couple of these moves. Even if you bypass the shower, still keep a towel around.

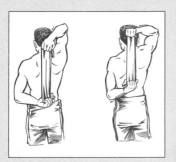

· Shoulder/Triceps Stretch: Drape the towel down the middle of your back, grabbing one end behind your neck and the other behind your lower back. Pull the top hand up for an internal rotator stretch, then pull the bottom hand down for a triceps and external rotator stretch. Do 5 slow reps of each, then switch hands.

· Chest Stretch: Fully extend your arm and wrap your palm around a stationary object, such as a doorjamb, at chest level. Turn your upper torso slowly until you feel a stretch in your chest muscle. Hold for a few seconds and release; repeat 4 times.

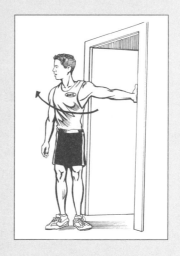

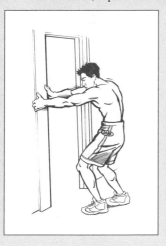

· Back Stretch: Bend your knees and grasp a stationary object, such as a doorjamb, in front of you at chest level. Lower your body as you extend your arms. Feel the stretch in your back for a few seconds, then release; repeat 4 times.

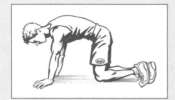
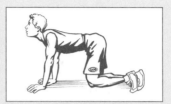

· Lower Back Stretch: Get down on your hands and knees. With your arms straight, slowly arch your back toward the sky while bringing your head and pelvis toward the floor (like a camel). When you reach the bottom of the stretch, arch your back toward the ground while lifting your head and pelvis up (like a cat). Do 3 sets of 5 reps each.

· Hip Flexors Stretch: With an erect torso, rest on your right knee, which should be directly under your hip. Your left leg is in front of you, bent at 90 degrees, and your left foot is flat on the ground. From that position, try to tuck your buttocks under your hips. Lean-ing forward only a couple of inches will give you the stretch you need. Hold for 10 seconds and repeat 3 times. Switch legs.

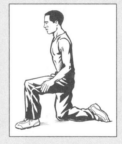
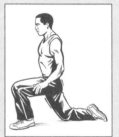

· Thigh Stretch: Remaining in the same position as above, reach behind to grasp your left ankle. Make sure your right ankle, knee, and hip are aligned parallel to the floor. Lean your torso forward and pull your left ankle toward your buttocks by flexing your hamstring until you feel the stretch in the quadriceps. Hold for a few seconds, then release. Lean forward with your hips (as the other leg supports you) to get a more ad-vanced stretch. Repeat 5 times, then switch sides.

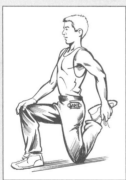

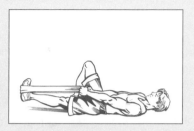
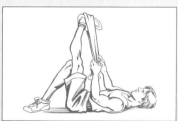

· Hamstring Stretch: Lie on your back. Bend your right leg and place that foot flat on the ground. Loop a towel around your left foot. Lock your left knee to keep your leg straight, then flex your quadriceps to lift your left leg as far up as you can from your hip. Aim your foot toward the ceiling. Grasp the ends of the towel with both hands and "climb" up the towel, hand over hand, as your leg lifts. Use the towel for gentle assistance at the end of the stretch. Stretch for only 2 seconds (before the muscle tightens up), then release. Repeat for a total of 10 reps, then switch sides.

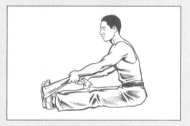
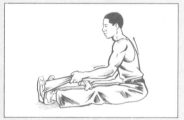

· Calf Stretch. Sit on the floor with both legs straight out in front of you. Loop the towel around your left foot and grasp each end of the towel in your hands. From your heel, flex your foot back toward your ankle, aiming your toes toward your knee. Use the towel for a gentle assist at the end of this movement. Again, hold the stretch for only 2 seconds, then release. Do 10 reps, then switch sides.

Week 1: Power

We're going to start off with a bang: this week's workout is geared toward packing on the muscle. As long as you take each set to complete muscle fatigue, your physique will be pushed to start growing now! The rest times may appear short, but I'm actually giving you more of a break than in the other weeks—so enjoy! Because you know that you have a rest coming after each set, don't hold back. Pick a weight where there's no way you could do another rep past the prescribed number.

- Do 3 sets of each exercise: 15, 12, and 10 reps (except for abs and lower back), and increase the weight as the reps decline for each set.

- Rest intervals: Rest for the amount of time it takes to change the weight, take five deep breaths, focus on what you're doing, and begin the next set.

▪ Monday and Thursday ▪

ABDOMINALS

2 trisets (3 exercises back-to-back-to-back without resting, then a short rest before starting over) of 15 reps each: Crossover Bicycle (page 69) + Reverse Crunch (page 69) + Long-Arm Crunch (page 70)

LOWER BACK

2 bisets (2 exercises back-to-back without resting, then a short rest before starting over) of 5 slow reps each: Straight-Leg Lift (page 70) + Upper Torso Lift (page 71)

CHEST

Flat Bench Press (page 71)
Dumbbell Flye (page 72)

SHOULDERS

Dumbbell Seated Military Press (page 73)
Dumbbell Side Lateral Raise (page 73)
Dumbbell External Rotator Flye (page 74)

TRICEPS

Incline Two-Dumbbell Triceps Extension (page 74)
Dumbbell Kickback (page 75)

▪ Tuesday and Friday ▪

LEGS

Squat (page 75)
Dumbbell Lunge (page 76)
Leg Curl (page 76)
One-Legged Calf Raise (page 77)

BACK

Wide-Grip Chin-up (maximum reps or chair-assisted) (page 77)
Dumbbell One-Arm Row (page 78)

BICEPS

Standing Barbell Curl (page 78)
Standing Dumbbell Hammer Curl (page 79)

Week 2: Stamina

Challenging your muscles to reach 13 reps or so with a weight that you normally can lift only 10 times is great, but this week you will go even further. After the initial 12 to 15 reps are done, you will take some weight off and grunt through another 10 reps or so. At that point, your muscles will be truly spent, with every muscle fiber hit. You will build size and strength with the first heavy load, then keep going with a lighter load to produce phenomenal endurance strength. Building this type of strength will give you great power, whether on the sports field, in the classroom, or in your future. Why? Because you will never get tired!

· Do 2 sets of each exercise: Start with a weight with which you can do only about 12 to 15 reps, then drop the weight down for another 10 reps.

· Rest intervals: Rest for the amount of time it takes to change the weight, take five deep breaths, focus on what you're doing, and begin the next set.

▪ Monday and Thursday ▪

ABDOMINALS

2 trisets of 20 reps each: Crossover Bicycle (page 69) + Reverse Crunch (page 69) + Long-Arm Crunch (page 70)

LOWER BACK

2 bisets of 8 slow reps each: Straight-Leg Lift (page 70) + Upper Torso Lift (page 71)

CHEST

Flat Bench Press (page 71)
Dumbbell Flye (page 72)

SHOULDERS

Dumbbell Seated Military Press (page 73)
Dumbbell Side Lateral Raise (page 73)
Dumbbell External Rotator Flye (page 74)

TRICEPS

Incline Two-Dumbbell Triceps Extension (page 74)
Dumbbell Kickback (page 75)

▪ Tuesday and Friday ▪

LEGS

Squat (page 75)
Dumbbell Lunge (page 76)
Leg Curl (page 76)
One-Legged Calf Raise (page 77)

BACK

Wide-Grip Chin-up (maximum reps or chair-assisted) (page 77)
Dumbbell One-Arm Row (page 78)

BICEPS

Standing Barbell Curl (page 78)
Standing Dumbbell Hammer Curl (page 79)

Exercise Descriptions for Weeks 1 and 2

▪ Crossover Bicycle ▪

Lie on your back with your hands clasped behind your head. Use a bicycle-pedaling motion with your legs, extending your left leg until it's almost straight while you bring your right knee up to your midsection. At the same time, bring your left shoulder off the ground and reach your left elbow toward your right knee. Alternate sides after every rep.

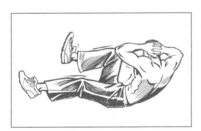 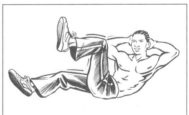

Jake Tip: Cup your hands behind your ears rather than behind your neck to eliminate neck strain.

▪ Reverse Crunch ▪

Lie on your back on a padded surface with your knees bent and your feet off the floor. Put your hands straight out to the sides. Flex your abs and begin pulling your pelvis up and toward your rib cage, moving slowly and exhaling at the same time. Continue until your abs are fully contracted and your hips are raised off the floor. Pause, continue to flex the abs, and breathe out any remaining air. Without releasing the tension of your abs, slowly lower to the start position.

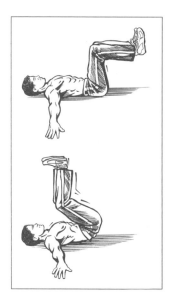

▪ Long-Arm Crunch ▪

Lie down on a padded surface with your shoulders and midback flat. Bend your legs and put your feet flat on the floor. Put your arms straight out behind you. Flex your abs and pull your rib cage up slowly, exhaling at the same time. Your arms come up with you, in line with your head and torso. Go until your abs are fully contracted, while your lower back remains firmly pressed against the floor. Pause, continue to flex the abs, and breathe out any remaining air. Without releasing the tension of your abs, slowly lower to the start position.

Jake Tip: Imagine that there is a tennis ball under your chin so you don't overflex your neck.

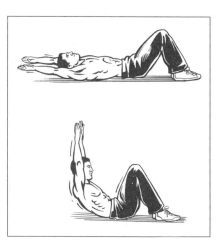

▪ Straight-Leg Lift ▪

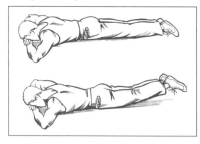

Lie facedown on a padded surface with your hands under your forehead, palms down. Firmly press your pelvis into the floor as you begin to raise your legs. Lift your legs by using your thigh muscles, and keep your knees locked. Feel your lower back, buttocks, and hamstrings contract as you bring your straight legs as high up as is comfortable. Hold, continue to contract your muscles, then slowly lower to the start position.

Jake Tip: If raising both legs is too difficult right now, do one leg at a time.

▪ Upper Torso Lift ▪

Lie facedown on a padded surface. Place your arms next to your sides. Raise your head and chest slightly off the floor to put tension on the lower back muscles. Flex the lower back and continue to raise your trunk. Pull your shoulder blades together and down toward your buttocks. Go to the point where your lower back is fully contracted without any spinal pain. Hold, continue to flex the lower back, then slowly lower to the start position.

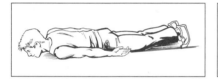 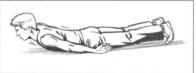

Jake Tip: Next month, graduate to cupping your ears with your hands.

▪ Flat Bench Press ▪

Lie on a flat bench with your knees bent and your feet flat on the floor. Keep a natural arch in your lower back and your buttocks on the bench for the entire exercise. Pull your shoulder blades together and hold them there throughout the exercise. Place your hands on the bar slightly wider than shoulder width apart and remove the barbell from the rack, grasping it in an overhand grip. Raise the barbell and hold it above your chest without locking your elbows. Slowly lower the weight to within a couple of inches of your chest, pause briefly, then press it back up to an extended position. Make sure that your lower back remains on the bench at all times.

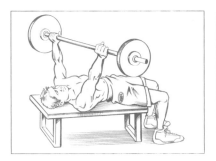 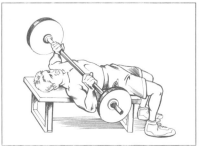

Jake Tip: You will see most guys bring the bar down to touch their chest, but your muscles and especially your shoulder joints will benefit from keeping it at least two inches above.

▪ Dumbbell Flye ▪

Sitting on the end of a bench with your feet flat on the floor, grasp a dumbbell in each hand and place one on each knee. Roll back as you bring your legs up to help put the dumbbells in the starting position, your arms extended upward with your elbows slightly bent. Pull your shoulder blades together and hold them there throughout the exercise. Keep a natural arch in your lower back and your buttocks on the bench for the entire exercise. Lower your arms outward until they're parallel to the ground. Hold, then flex the chest, and then pull your arms up and together to the start position. Keep your chest tight at the finish of each rep.

Jake Tip: Keep the dumbbells over your lower rib cage instead of your chest to hit more of the muscle.

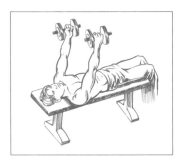 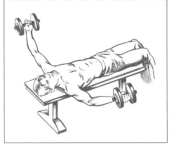

▪ Dumbbell Seated Military Press ▪

Sit upright on a bench with your feet shoulder width apart and your torso erect. Grasp the dumbbells in an overhand grip. Bring the dumbbells to a parallel position with your ears, your palms facing forward. Pull your shoulder blades together and hold them there throughout the exercise. Flex your shoulders, then push the weights overhead and together without locking your elbows. Pause briefly and slowly lower the weight back to the starting position.

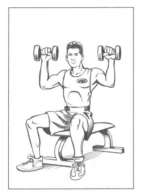 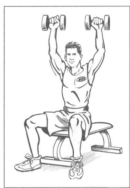

Jake Tip: Keeping the dumbbells on the same plane as your chest, rather than in front of your head or especially behind the head, will get rid of any potential shoulder strain.

▪ Dumbbell Side Lateral Raise ▪

Stand with your feet shoulder width apart. Grasp a dumbbell in each hand. Slightly bend your knees and lean forward at the waist. With your arms hanging straight down and your palms facing each other, look straight ahead. Maintaining a stable torso, contract your shoulders as you bring your straight arms

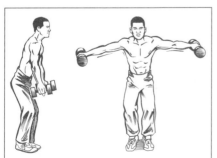

out to the sides to just below shoulder level. Hold, continue to contract your shoulders, then slowly lower your arms to the start position.

Jake Tip: Resist the tendency to swing the dumbbells to assist each rep.

▪ Dumbbell External Rotator Flye ▪

Lie down on your side. Hold a light weight (such as a 2.5-pound plate or 5-pound DB) in your top hand with your arm in a 90-degree angle on top of your hip, holding the weight in front of you on the floor. Press your upper arm tightly against the side of your body, flex the back of your shoulder, and rotate the weight from the ground in a semicircle until your hand points to the sky. Return to the start position. Switch sides after completing half the set.

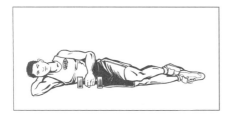 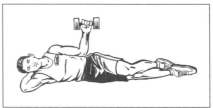

Jake Tip: Keep your hand relaxed and instead feel only the back of your shoulder working.

▪ Incline Two-Dumbbell Triceps Extension ▪

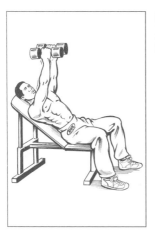 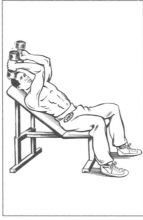

Set your bench at a high incline. Place your shoulder blades and head firmly against the bench. Position your arms straight up with your elbows slightly bent. Slowly lower your forearms, without moving your shoulders or upper arms, until your arms form a 90-degree angle and the dumbbells are on either side of your face. Hold, continue to flex your triceps, and slowly push the dumbbells back up.

Jake Tip: Keep a slight bend in your elbows as you finish each rep to keep the pressure on the muscle rather than the joint.

▪ Dumbbell Kickback ▪

Place your right knee in the center of the bench, with your left foot nearby on the floor and your left knee slightly bent. Place your right hand on the bench in front of your shoulder with your back parallel to the floor. Pick up a dumbbell in your left hand. Turn your palm in, bend your elbow, and hold the weight by your side. Relax your shoulder, and keep your shoulder blades squeezed together. Slowly extend your arm backward until the weight is parallel to the ground. Keep your elbow anchored to your side. Switch sides after completing half the set.

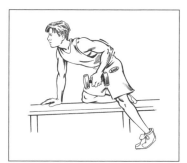 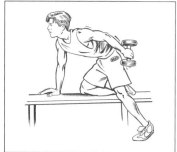

Jake Tip: Use a slow rep speed rather than momentum to push the weight back up.

▪ Squat ▪

Standing, hold a barbell behind your neck and across your trapezius muscles. Straighten your legs to lift the bar off the rack and move back a step. Place your feet shoulder width apart, toes angled slightly outward. Keep your upper-body muscles rigid, your torso slightly leaning forward, and a natural arch in your lower back. Focus on a spot on the wall slightly above eye level. Bend your hips and knees while smoothly descending to a point where your thighs are parallel to the ground, as if you were sitting in a chair. Flex your

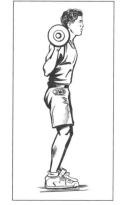 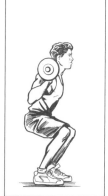

thigh, buttock, and hamstring muscles, then push back up to the top position without locking your knees.

Jake Tip: Keep the weight centered over your ankles throughout
the exercise.

▪ Dumbbell Lunge ▪

Stand erect while holding the dumbbells down at your sides. Keep your pelvis and hips level. Take a large step forward with one leg and land softly on your heel, keeping your pelvis directly under your shoulders. Lower yourself until your forward thigh is parallel to the floor, with your torso still leaning slightly forward. Flex your thigh, buttocks, and hamstring muscles, then push back up to start position. Alternate sides after each rep.

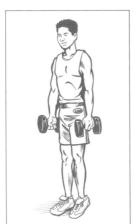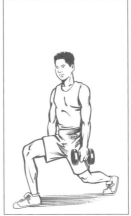

Jake Tip: Your forward knee should never go beyond the vertical plane
of your forward toes.

▪ Leg Curl ▪

Lie face down on the bench with your knee joints just over the front end. Put your heels just beyond the pad. Grasp the sides of the bench. Begin with your knees slightly flexed. Contract your hamstrings and pull your lower legs up slowly, keeping your pelvis pressed down and lifting the knees only slightly above the bench. Pull your heels until they almost reach your buttocks, and

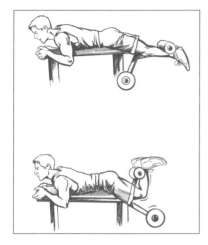

continue to flex your hamstrings while you relax your feet. Slowly lower your legs down to the start position. (If you don't have a leg curl apparatus, use a dynamic tension band: loop one end of the band around your left ankle and the other end around your right foot. Stand up straight and hold on to a stable object for balance. Curl your left heel upward toward your buttocks while flexing your hamstring muscle. Try to keep your working knee in the same place throughout the movement. Switch legs after each set.)

Jake Tip: With the apparatus, occasionally do one-legged leg curls to make sure one side isn't taking more of the weight.

▪ One-Legged Calf Raise ▪

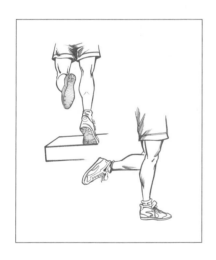

Hold a dumbbell at the side of your right leg. Place the ball of your right foot on a step or stair, pointing the foot straight forward. With your left hand, hold on to something for balance. Contract your right calf muscle and raise your right heel until your ankle is fully extended. Keep a natural bend in your knee. Pause in the top position, then lower until your right heel is just below your toes on the step. Switch legs after each set.

Jake Tip: For every rep, aim for a full contraction at the top for maximum development.

▪ Wide-Grip Chin-up ▪

Grasp an overhead bar in an overhand grip with your hands more than shoulder width apart. Begin with your arms fully extended and slightly bent. If you need assistance, put a chair under you so the top of your feet can rest on

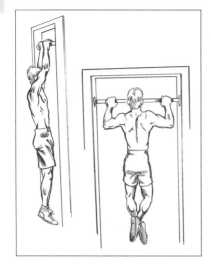

it and take some of the weight. Pull your shoulder blades down and together, and maintain a natural arch in your back. Flex your outer back (or lateral) muscles, and pull your elbows out as your body comes up. Pull up until your chin is positioned above the bar. Pause, lower, and repeat.

Jake Tip: Do not allow your shoulders to hunch forward at the last part of the rep.

▪ Dumbbell One-Arm Row ▪

Place your left knee in the center of a bench with your right foot nearby on the floor and your right knee slightly bent. Place your left hand on the bench in front of your shoulder with your back parallel to the floor. Lightly hold the dumbbell with your arm hanging straight down, keeping your shoulder blades back. Pull your arm up with your elbow pointing straight back and close to your body. Flex your upper back and maintain a natural arch in your lower back. Return to the start position. Switch sides after half the set.

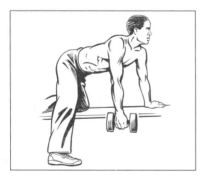
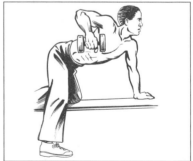

Jake Tip: Keep a relaxed arm and hand so the dumbbell is lifted mostly by your back, not your biceps.

▪ Standing Barbell Curl ▪

Stand with your knees slightly bent, your feet shoulder width apart. Hold a barbell at waist level in an underhand grip with your hands shoulder width apart. Start with the bar resting against the front of your thighs and your elbows at your sides. Flex your biceps as you curl the barbell to your chest. Pause briefly at the top, then slowly lower to the starting position.

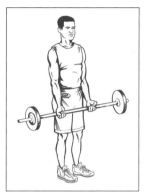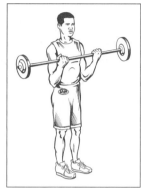

Jake Tip: Keep your torso upright and your elbows anchored to your sides to keep the tension on your biceps constant.

▪ Standing Dumbbell Hammer Curl ▪

Stand with your feet shoulder width apart. Hold the dumbbells in front of your thighs so your palms face each other. Anchor your elbows to your sides. Contract your biceps and curl both dumbbells upward in front of your body. Raise the dumbbells as far as they will go without moving your upper arms.

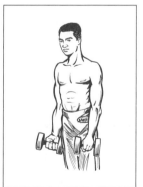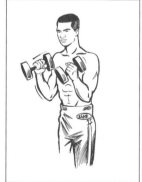

Jake Tip: Extend dumbbells down as far as your biceps will let you without taking pressure off the muscle.

Week 3: Strength

The endurance strength training continues this week, although this time each muscle group is trained using supersets, which add additional muscle shaping. A superset involves doing two exercises for the same muscle back-to-back without a rest period. Because you're doing two exercises in a short time frame, more of your muscle is affected than with the typical one-exercise approach. While you won't have as much energy to give to the second exercise, I've put the less-tough exercise in that place so that your superset's second half should still almost equal the first half in intensity!

· Do a superset of two exercises for each body part: 3 supersets for each body part; 20 reps total for the superset, or 10 reps for each exercise.

· Rest interval: Rest for the amount of time it takes to change the weight for both exercises, take five deep breaths, focus on what you're doing, and begin the next set.

· If a regular push-up is too difficult, do it on your knees. Too easy? Elevate your feet to a bench or chair, but make sure your body still forms a straight line from ankle to head.

▪ Monday and Thursday ▪

ABDOMINALS

3 trisets of 20 reps each: Vertical-Leg Crunch (page 83) + Leg Lift (page 84) + Side-to-Side Crunch (page 84)

LOWER BACK

3 bisets of 10 slow reps each: Superman (page 85) + Alternate Lying Hyperextension (page 85)

CHEST

Dumbbell Incline Press (page 85)
Wide-Stance Push-up (page 86)

SHOULDERS

Standing Military Press (page 87)

Alternate Dumbbell Front Shoulder Raise (page 87)

Dumbbell Internal Rotator Flye (page 88): Do 2 straight sets of 12 to 15 reps each.

TRICEPS

Lying Dumbbell French Press (page 88)

One-Arm Dumbbell Overhead Triceps Extension (page 89)

▪ Tuesday and Friday ▪

LEGS

Dumbbell Strider Squat (page 89)

Lunge (page 90)

Leg Curl (page 76): Superset the leg curl and calf raise even though they're different muscle groups.

One-Legged Calf Raise (page 77)

BACK

Bent-Over Row (page 90)

Close-Grip, Underhand Pull-up (page 91)

BICEPS

Standing Dumbbell Rotating Curl (page 91)

One-Arm Dumbbell Preacher Curl (page 92)

Week 4: Super Stamina and Strength

In the final workout week of the month, it makes sense to work on your reserves. You want to be the guy who always has something extra at the end, whether in your sport, your summer job, or your exam. These monster sets expand your energy tank by not flooring it off the starting line this time around. Instead, the first 10 reps are executed with a weight that you're still strong with at rep 10. Then you hold the weight at extension—being careful not to lock your joints—for five counts. This will take a little more strength out of you, and then you hit it hard for another 10 reps. By this point, the next hold and following miniset will be pure guts. If you can't do 10 reps in the third round, that's okay. But try for as many as possible. This week will open your eyes even more to what kind of physical level you can go to; your mind will join you every step of the way.

· 2 monster sets of each exercise: Each monster set consists of 10 reps. Then you hold the weight at extension for 5 seconds, then immediately do another 10 reps, then hold again for 5 seconds, then 10 more reps, for a total of 30 reps.

· Rest interval: Rest for the amount of time it takes to change the weight for the exercise, take five deep breaths, focus on what you're doing, and begin the next set.

▪ Monday and Thursday ▪

ABDOMINALS

3 trisets of 25 reps each: Vertical-Leg Crunch (page 83) + Leg Lift (page 84) + Side-to-Side Crunch (page 84)

LOWER BACK

3 bisets of 12 slow reps each: Superman (page 85) + Alternate Lying Hyperextension (page 85)

CHEST

Dumbbell Incline Press (page 86)
Wide-Stance Push-up (page 86)

SHOULDERS

Standing Military Press (page 87)
Alternate Dumbbell Front Shoulder Raise (page 87)
Dumbbell Internal Rotator Flye (page 88): 3 straight sets of 12 to 15 reps

TRICEPS

Lying Dumbbell French Press (page 88)
One-Arm Dumbbell Overhead Triceps Extension (page 89)

▪ Tuesday and Friday ▪

LEGS

Dumbbell Strider Squat (page 89)
Lunge (page 90)
Leg Curl (page 76)
One-Legged Calf Raise (page 77)

BACK

Bent-Over Row (page 90)
Close-Grip, Underhand Pull-up (page 91)

BICEPS

Standing Dumbbell Rotating Curl (page 91)
One-Arm Dumbbell Preacher Curl (page 92)

New Exercise Descriptions for Weeks 3 and 4

▪ Vertical-Leg Crunch ▪

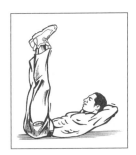

Lie on your back, bend your knees slightly, and raise your legs so your thighs are perpendicular to the floor. Cup your hands behind your head, then flex your abs and pull your rib cage up slowly, exhaling at the same time. Go until your abs are fully contracted, while your lower back remains firmly pressed against the floor. Hold, continue to flex your abs, and breathe out any remaining air. Without releasing the tension of your abs, slowly lower to the start position.

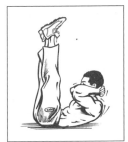

Jake Tip: If you find it difficult to keep your legs straight, cross them at the ankles.

▪ Leg Lift ▪

Sit on the end of a bench and brace yourself by holding the bench's sides behind you. Begin with your legs tucked into your chest. Straighten them on a slight angle toward the ground, then flex your ab and hip muscles as you pull your legs slowly in to your chest.

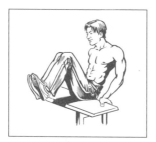 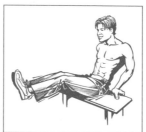

Jake Tip: Keep your torso as stable as possible to focus the movement on your abs.

▪ Side-to-Side Crunch ▪

Lie on your back with your right knee bent and right foot flat on the floor. Cross your left ankle over your right knee. Press your lower back into the floor and bring your right hand behind your right ear. Contract your abs and side muscles, then slowly curl your right shoulder up toward your left knee. Hold briefly and lower to the start position. Switch sides after half the set.

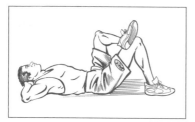 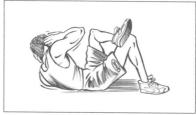

Jake Tip: Put your hand on the working side of your abs to feel the muscles contract during every rep.

▪ Superman ▪

Lie facedown on a padded surface with your arms in front of you. Put your legs together with the top part of your feet resting on the mat. Firmly press your

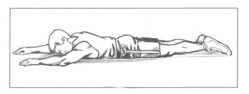

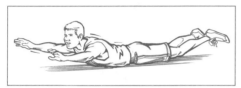

pelvis into the floor as you flex your lower back and simultaneously raise your legs and upper body. Lift your legs by using your thigh muscles, and pull your shoulder blades together until you achieve full contraction. Hold, then lower to the start position.

Jake Tip: **Keep your head aligned with your trunk at all times.**

▪ Alternate Lying Hyperextension ▪

Lie facedown on a padded surface with your arms in front of you. Put your legs together with the top part of your feet resting on the mat. Firmly press your pelvis into the floor as you flex your lower back and simultaneously raise

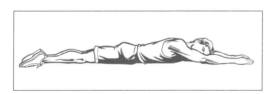

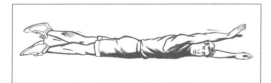

your left leg and right arm and shoulder off the ground. Lift your leg by using your thigh muscle, and pull your shoulder blades together until you achieve full contraction. Hold, then lower to the start position. Alternate sides after half the set.

Jake Tip: **Don't overhyperextend; instead, just go to the point where you feel your muscle is fully flexed.**

▪ Dumbbell Incline Press ▪

Set the incline board at about 45 degrees. Lean back on the bench. Plant your feet firmly on the floor and keep a natural arch in your lower back. Pull your shoulder blades together and hold them there throughout the exercise. Bring dumbbells from on top of your knees to their start position: poised above your chest. Flex your chest as you push the dumbbells vertically up from your chest until your arms are almost straight. Slowly bring them back down to the start position.

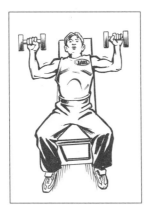 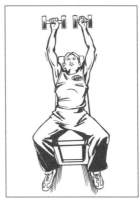

Jake Tip: Keep your lower back in contact with the bench at all times.

▪ Wide-Stance Push-up ▪

Position your head, torso, hips, and knees in a straight line. Place your hands slightly wider than chest width apart. Maintain a slight arch in your lower back. Pull your shoulder blades together and hold them there throughout the exercise. Press up to the starting position, with a slight bend in your elbows. Descend until your arms form 90-degree angles and your elbows bend out to the sides. Hold and contract the chest, then push back up to the start position.

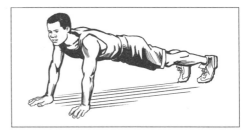

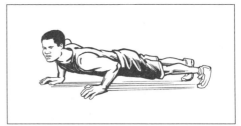

Jake Tip: To take the stress off your wrists, turn your hands slightly inward and keep your weight on the heels of your hands.

▪ Standing Military Press ▪

Stand upright with your knees slightly bent and your feet flat on the floor, shoulder width apart. Grasp a barbell in an overhand grip, bend your elbows, and hold it in front of your eyes. Pull your shoulder blades together and hold them there throughout the exercise. Flex your shoulders, then raise the barbell overhead vertically in alignment with your chest without locking your elbows. Pause briefly and slowly lower the weight back to the starting position.

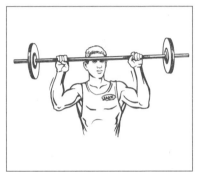 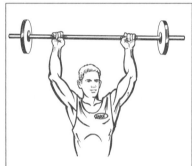

Jake Tip: Never bring the bar behind your neck, as that position can damage your shoulder joints.

▪ Alternate Dumbbell Front Shoulder Raise ▪

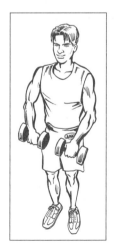 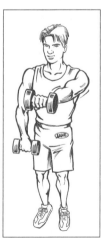

Stand with your feet shoulder width apart. Slightly bend your knees and hips. Hold a dumbbell in each hand with your arms straight and your palms against your thighs. Begin with the arms slightly forward so there's tension on the front shoulder muscles. Flex these muscles as you raise your left arm up and slightly out. Keep your elbow pointing down. Pause at shoulder height, then slowly bring the dumbbell back down to the start position. Alternate sides after each rep.

Jake Tip: Relax your hands and arms in order to keep the tension on the shoulder muscles.

▪ Dumbbell Internal Rotator Flye ▪

Lie down on your side on the floor. Hold a dumbbell in the bottom hand, with your arm forming a 90-degree angle and your upper arm perpendicular to your body. Keep your head and neck in a neutral position. Begin with the dumbbell just off the floor. Flex the front part of your shoulder and rotate the dumbbell up until it points to the sky. Slowly return to the start position.

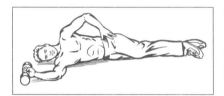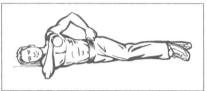

Jake Tip: This exercise is designed to strengthen the tiny rotator cuff muscles. Therefore, keep the weight on the light side, about 2.5 to 5 pounds.

▪ Lying Dumbbell French Press ▪

Grasp a dumbbell in each hand. Lie down on a bench with your knees bent and your feet flat on the floor. Maintain a natural arch in your lower back. Keep your upper arms and elbows stationary. Extend your arms toward the ceiling. Then lower the dumbbells toward your head as your elbows point toward the ceiling, forming a 90-degree angle. Flex your triceps as you push back to a straight-arm position.

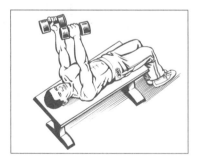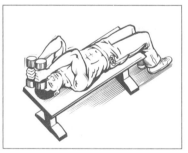

Jake Tip: Keep the weights over your head and not behind, because that is the perfect action to strengthen the triceps.

▪ One-Arm Dumbbell Overhead Triceps Extension ▪

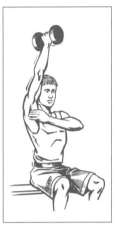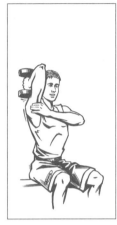

Sit upright on a bench with your knees bent, feet on the floor. Holding a dumbbell in your right hand, extend your right arm straight up with your elbow slightly bent. Slowly lower the dumbbell to a 90-degree angle just behind your head. Keep your right shoulder and upper arm still. Flex your triceps and slowly push the dumbbell back up. Switch sides after half the set.

Jake Tip: Try to have your working elbow point at the sky throughout the move.

▪ Dumbbell Strider Squat ▪

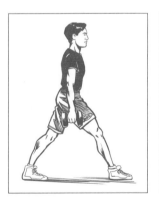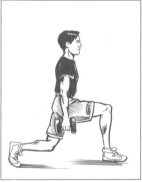

Standing, hold a dumbbell at each side. Step forward with your right foot about three feet and position your torso so it is about one foot behind your right foot. Lean your torso slightly forward and maintain a natural arch in your lower back. Drop your buttocks straight down until your right thigh is parallel to the ground. Your left heel will come off the ground. Pause briefly, then flex your thighs, buttocks, and hamstring muscles as you push yourself back up to the start position. Switch sides after half the set.

Jake Tip: Allow your front leg to carry more of the load than the back.

▪ Lunge ▪

Stand erect, holding a barbell across the back of your shoulders. Keep your pelvis and hips level. Take a large step forward with your left foot, landing softly on your heel and keeping your pelvis directly under your shoulders. Lower yourself until your left thigh is parallel to the floor, with your torso still leaning slightly forward. Flex your thigh, buttocks, and hamstring muscles, then push back up to the start position. Alternate sides after each rep.

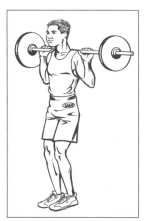 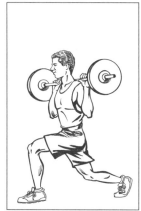

Jake Tip: Push explosively back to the start position for extra leg power.

▪ Bent-Over Row ▪

Stand with your feet shoulder width apart. Grasp a barbell with an overhand grip just beyond shoulder width. Hold it down at arm's length. Bend your knees, then bend from your waist and lean your trunk down about 45 degrees.

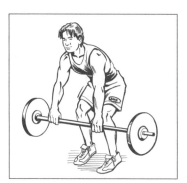 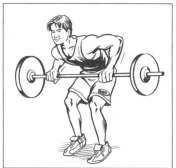

Pull your shoulder blades together and maintain a natural arch in your lower back. Flex your upper back muscles and pull the bar straight up to around your ribs, keeping your elbows close to your sides. Pause briefly, then lower to the start position.

> **Jake Tip:** To keep from rounding your back during this exercise, lift your head up and look straight ahead as you pull up the weight.

■ Close-Grip, Underhand Pull-up ■

Grasp an overhead bar with an underhand grip with your hands a little less than shoulder width apart. If you need assistance, put a chair under your 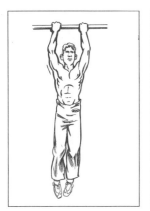 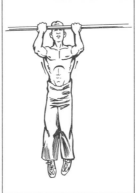 feet so they can rest on it and take some of the weight. Begin with your arms fully extended and slightly bent. Pull your shoulder blades down and together, maintaining a natural arch in your back. Flex your lats and pull your elbows out as your body comes up. Pull up until your chin is positioned above the bar. Pause, lower, and repeat.

> **Jake Tip:** Try to relax your arms in order to make your back, not your biceps, do most of the work.

■ Standing Dumbbell Rotating Curl ■

Stand with your knees slightly bent. Hold a dumbbell at each side with your palms facing in. Keep your elbows anchored to your sides. Flex your biceps as you slowly rotate the weights upward until your palms are outside your shoulders, facing backward. Pause briefly, then slowly lower the weights to the start position.

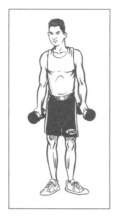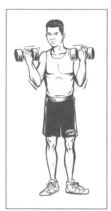

Jake Tip: Although you turn your wrists as you bring the weight up,
don't bend your wrists.

▪ One-Arm Dumbbell Preacher Curl ▪

Position one arm down the middle of an incline board as you take an athletic stance behind the bench. Holding a dumbbell with your arm flexed,
slowly let it down until your arm is almost straight. Pause, then contract your
biceps and curl the dumbbell back to the start position. Switch sides after half
the set.

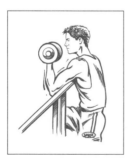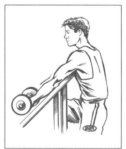

Jake Tip: Keep your wrists in line with your forearm to take pressure
off the joint.

MONTH 2 AND BEYOND

Now you're ready to add more volume to your larger muscle groups, so add one exercise for your chest, thighs, and back. Since month 2 represents about the perfect training amount for your body, month 3 and beyond can follow the same pattern, as long as you switch the exercises around every new week. Crank it up!

WEEK 5, POWER: Do 3 sets of each exercise (12, 10, 8 reps), adding more weight for each set.

WEEK 6, STAMINA: Do 3 sets of each exercise: start with 10 to 12 reps, then drop down for another 5 to 8 reps.

WEEK 7, STRENGTH: Do a triset of three exercises for chest, thighs, and back; a superset of two exercises for the rest of the body; do 3 trisets or supersets for each body part of 8 to 10 reps for each exercise (24 to 30 total reps for each triset; 16 to 20 total reps for each superset).

WEEK 8, SUPER STAMINA AND STRENGTH: Do 2 monster sets of each exercise, with each monster set consisting of 8 to 10 reps, then hold the weight at extension for 5 seconds, then immediately do another 8 to 10 more reps, then hold again for 5 seconds, then do 8 to 10 more reps for 24 to 30 total reps.

Powerful men and women throughout history have been told that they were "born leaders." Of these, however, the great majority achieved success by sheer effort and personality, whatever the circumstances of their birth. You're born rich or poor, black or white, but you don't become a leader unless you work hard earning your stripes.

Granted, sometimes you're born into a situation where leadership is called for more often—such as being born the oldest, as I was—but it remains in your hands to actually develop the skills. I know my two little brothers looked up to me during most of my youth for one reason: I was older. It wasn't until later in my teenage years that I gradually became a genuine leader for them.

Why am I going on about being a leader? Simple: if you want to achieve your goals and realize your dreams, being a leader is the only way to go. Chances are, though, that you are more of a follower right now. It's difficult not to be, since you and all your peers basically live the same routine day after day: getting up at a certain time, going to class all day, then engaging in an extracurricular activity like sports practice or a club meeting, then returning home, where you have dinner with your family, do your homework, and hit the sack. Did we forget something there? Hmm, maybe the goals and dreams that you woke up with? By nightfall, they lie crushed by the daily grind, just as your face gets lost in the crowd when you travel on the same road as everybody else.

It is time to break away from the herd. No, I don't mean skipping school and doing whatever you want with your day. I'm talking about becoming a leader—at school, with your friends, on the sports team, in the classroom, even in your family. Every day.

Do you see the connection between leading and achieving your goals? Maybe you'd like to have a diverse group of friends, so instead of flocking to a social group that you want to be a part of, create your own group! Maybe you long to become a great writer—ask your English teacher to recommend books beyond what you and your classmates are already reading. Perhaps you want your family to be closer—become the catalyst for doing more activities together.

In order to accomplish those kinds of things and become that sort of leader, you must have self-confidence. Until that self-confidence is there, your leadership as well as your grasp on your goals will be shaky at best. Many things and certain people around you may deter you from possessing the confidence and courage needed to carry out your goals, but who is it who permits those obstacles to stop you from taking what is rightly yours? You! Remember: nobody limits how good a shape you can be in, how successful, how smart . . . except yourself.

If you really want certain things, you'll be a leader and get them on your own, in your own way. That takes guts! Doing my workout four times a week, every week, is not easy; calling up your crush when you're not sure she even knows who you are isn't either, but you'll succeed if you take these steps.

Doing my workout may be the first time that you don't follow anyone else. You're training just for you, and you will discover something remarkable: that you can be a leader if you want to be one, and you can do whatever you want if you don't stand around looking for others to go first. There are some potential stumbling blocks along the way that you need to prepare for, however, before you take that lead. Get ready to take them on!

▪ Obstacles Are Actually Opportunities! ▪

You know that guy guarding you in a pickup game—the one who trash-talks you during every trip down the floor? He's an obstacle. You're going to have to get past him physically and mentally to score points and, hopefully, get him to stop running his mouth!

An obstacle is anyone or anything that keeps you from achieving your goals and doesn't go away easily! We all face apparently immovable obstacles—like your father dictating which college he wants you to attend—but most are in our heads. Take that guy in the pickup game, for instance: he isn't really much of a physical obstacle, but if you let him get to you, he could shut you down anyway.

My stuttering was a real obstacle, because it kept me from delivering a smooth speech in class or a smooth line to a cute girl! However, it grew into a massive head game: I'd think "don't stutter" way before I'd even open my mouth. I was a pretty confident guy, but my stuttering had begun to eat away at my confidence. And the few shreds of confidence I had left were being gobbled up by my overweight physique and big appetite! The things I wanted most as a young teenager—getting admiring looks and being a great basketball player—seemed unattainable due to my poor physical condition. As the rejections piled up, the pounds piled on. In my mind, I began to see myself as just a chubby kid and didn't think twice about going for seconds every day at lunch.

One day I realized that I had a choice: I could be overwhelmed by my obstacles of stuttering and chubbyhood, or I could go to the source of all the misery—my head—and reverse the trends. Training made that possible. In my basement I said good-bye to my fat and hello to a new, confident guy who wasn't going to stumble over his words, no matter what the situation. It was a tough process but one in which I began to see improvements, week by week.

You probably have some stubborn obstacles of your own. Triumph over them by training hard and plotting your course beyond them. That's what a leader does. Look at our most recent "leaders of the free world." Bill Clinton had an alcoholic father and George W. Bush had some trouble with alcohol as a young man—but they managed to become the most powerful men in America!

If anything, consider your obstacles as opportunities to make your future a more powerful one. If I hadn't started out fat and stuttering, I sincerely doubt I would have trained as hard in the gym or worked as hard in my business to make sure those obstacles never returned!

MUSCLE MAKER: *Channel Your Aggression*

Some of the obstacles you encounter may motivate you. They may also anger you. You can't seem to get an A in your Spanish class no matter how hard you try, or your nemesis is dating your favorite girl. Don't go out and tag your teacher's car or challenge your nemesis to a fight. You'll never get ahead that way. Instead, channel that aggression into your workout, where you can turn negative energy against somebody or something else into positive energy for yourself.

You're going to face tough times; you will receive some low blows; everyone does eventually. How you respond shows what kind of leader you are. You can sit in the gutter and focus on your problems there, but then you'll be stuck in that gutter. Instead, take your problems to your workout and watch them evaporate (along with all your sweat)! By the end of the session, your problems will seem either pretty insignificant or very conquerable. Your mind will be focused and positive. Plus, if you can crank through 360 reps for your chest, shoulders, and triceps in twenty minutes during Week 4, then you can accomplish anything!

▪ Get Out of the Box ▪

Without knowing it, you are put into boxes by people all the time. And the box is one of the fiercest obstacles, because it surrounds you on every side! From the time you're little, you're told what you can and can't do. Your parents tell you what you're good at and what you're not; your guidance counselor tells you which colleges you can get into and which ones you can't; your coach tells you which playing position you're suited for and which ones you're not.

Listen to those voices, and you'll end up kicking yourself later in life—I guarantee you! "I knew I should have gone into computers instead of law!" "I wanted to attend Columbia and probably would have been accepted, but just never applied." "I had the talent and arm to play quarterback, but got stuck playing tight end instead." Woulda, coulda, shoulda! Instead, listen to the voice inside your head. You know your dreams better than anyone; you know the great things you are capable of.

Your peers may convince you otherwise, however, because the box rarely gets smaller and sealed tighter than at school. Maybe you're the "jokester," the "jock," the "hippie," the "nerd"—and maybe it's been that way since grade school. The others expect you to always act the same way and look the same way. The danger is that often you find yourself falling into the trap and doing just that! You feel obligated to stay true to the stereotype. You, the hippie, doesn't think it's a big deal to smoke pot after school, or you, the jock, feel as if it's okay if you don't study. You end up helping other people build your box and hurting yourself!

REALITY CHECK: *Boxing Myself In—Temporarily!*

Some boxes that people put you into are actually well intentioned. My parents' strong expectation that I go to college was such a box. Everybody else's kid went to college, so why not me? As a result, I had the board and hammer ready to go when I faced the special admissions committee at Cortland State.

Because I hadn't scored high enough on the college entrance exams for regular admission, I had a shot through an admission program that admitted a few students who didn't meet academic standards, yet showed potential because of their leadership abilities or unique talents. In fact, my high school guidance counselor, Tommy Lamandola—who was also a bodybuilder and a role model for me—was the one who recommended me to this committee. He probably had a gut feeling that college wasn't the place for me, but what kind of guidance counselor would tell me that!

It certainly was my gut feeling, but there I sat in the backseat of my parents' car, headed to the Cortland State campus. Actually, I crouched back there when we arrived because I didn't want any of the students to see me in my one suit: a green corduroy beauty that was the perfect outfit for a hot, humid summer day. Dressing for success was one lesson I hadn't yet learned! Fortunately, I knew how to tap into my imagination. That Office of Admissions became Las Vegas in my mind, while the admissions committee was the audience. Me? The entertainment, of course.

When I heard my name called, I strode into the room and introduced myself to everyone, making eye contact and shaking everyone's hands. My model was my grandmother, Myra Duberstein, who could turn any stranger into a buddy in minutes. She had shown me how to work a crowd, and shown me well. "How ya doin'? I'm Jake Steinfeld, pleased to meetcha!" We sat down around a table the size of a Vegas stage, and the formal interview began. They explained the program to me and told me that more than a hundred other applicants were being considered—in case I didn't know the kind of pressure I was under. I knew! I opened my act with a joke. Most of them smiled; a few of them looked a bit shocked. Tough crowd. They hadn't heard my best material yet, however: "I think I can make Cortland State a better place. I like people. I'm a hard worker, and now that I've learned how to build my body, I think I can apply it to my studies. What can I say? I'm a late bloomer, but I think Cortland State can really help me grow and flourish. I'm willing to work hard if you give me the chance."

They bought it—hook, line, and sinker. All the committee members slapped me on the back and told me that I'd definitely be hearing from them soon. A few weeks later, I got the acceptance letter in the mail. I wanted to cry—and not tears of joy. Months later, I was cooped up in my little dorm room, trying to study—yep, stuck in a box! A box that I had helped erect, which made it all the more difficult to escape from.

In fact, when I gave my parents the big news—that I wanted to leave college and move to L.A. to become a bodybuilder—they didn't exactly burst with pride. However, I have to give my parents credit, because after a lot of convincing, they treated me like the adult that I wasn't. They saw my commitment to and excitement about my new goal and supported me, even if it meant my abandoning a higher education.

I was the "pudgy stutterer," so the last person anyone expected to volunteer to give a speech in class or speak up in the huddle was me. Meanwhile, everybody expected me to tote Twinkies in my backpack along with my books. Once I started training, slimming down, and becoming more confident, however, things began to change. I even started to look for opportunities to test the new confident Jake, minus the stutter. That meant talking in class more, introducing myself to people I didn't know, talking with adults more. Sure enough, my stutter started to fade. Talking to my teammates became so easy that I became team captain my sophomore year!

It's time for you to break out of your box, no matter what it is. If others and/or you don't think you can build muscle, improve your grades, or find a nice girlfriend, you're going to change that now! Training is the first getaway route, because you'll never look or feel the same again. Soon other people will notice the great changes in you as well. No one, especially yourself, will make the mistake of boxing you up ever again!

STUMBLING . . . TO SUCCESS: No More Teasing This Teenage Guy!

Not everyone will accept the new you, however. After losing about 15 pounds of fat while jacking his bench press to more than 300 pounds, seventeen-year-old Zack Harper got plenty of encouraging comments from his family, friends, and football coaches. However, one guy who liked him as

"Fat Zack" wasn't so happy and one day actually started razzing him more than before—first at school, then even at the gym. Zack's first thought was to go kick his butt, but after some good advice from a friend, he choose to show him on the football field. Two days later, Zack nearly took this guy's head off with a tackle during practice. Guess what? He hasn't heard a peep from that clown since.

There will be people, mostly peers, who show their jealousy in different ways after you start making great changes. Just as your training is responsible for those changes, it can also serve as a cushion against the verbal blows (or even physical, if it comes to that) you may face. Instead of letting them get to you, feel sorry for those folks!

▪ Fear: Stare It Down and Walk Right Past It ▪

While obstacles and boxes can slow or halt your progress, fear can prevent you from even getting started. "I'm so skinny that everyone at the gym will make fun of me. I think I'll skip it." Or "I'm sure she's got a boyfriend, so why bother go up and say hello?" Sound familiar? That's fear getting the best of you.

Fear gets a head start in childhood, when it's the primitive fear of being abandoned by our parents, the dark, deep water, and so on. When you bought into those fears, you gave them power by creating some kind of monster. As a teenager, the same process occurs, but this time the sources of your fears are different: rejection, criticism, and responsibility, among others.

Often these fears can be crippling; for example, you may never take on any challenges because you imagine being rejected or criticized. Maybe you fear loneliness, so you always have to have a girlfriend or friends around you. The situation can worsen to the point that your fears begin to control your actions, rather than you taking action to get over your fears!

Just as when you, as a kid, learned that there is not a monster in your closet, as a teenager you can realize that your fears are often just your imagination running in the wrong direction. You can have well-defined goals and the perfect plan to go after them, along with plenty of love and support from the right people, but they can all be derailed by fear. Waking up from a nightmare makes it come to an abrupt close; learning to see fear as a temporary emotion can erase it just as quickly.

POWER HABIT: *Challenge Fear Whenever It Appears*

Fear is often regarded as an emotion without benefit, but it actually has many things to teach you about yourself. If you face it with the right frame of mind, you will not only overcome it but grow as a person.

1. *Characterize your fear.* Are you afraid of failure or success? Are you worried about what others will say or think about you if you fail? Or do you think you won't be able to handle success? Nail down exactly what your fear is and tell yourself that you can beat it! Understanding the enemy is half the battle.

2. *Go straight at that fear.* Don't run away from it, and don't try to go around it. You only go backward when you shy away from fear, because doing so gives it more ammunition. However, successfully confronting it builds up a store of confidence that will allow you to do the same the next time around. Even when something doesn't work out, remind yourself that the majority of the time, you, and not fear, will prevail!

3. *Let fear energize you.* When you feel fear taking over, learn to find the "energy outlet" inside you. Recognize fear as a natural instinct that is simply preparing you to face a challenge. It can serve a positive purpose, rather than a negative one, once you discover that outlet. Nervous about scoring in the big game? Turn up your defense, and your offense will come naturally. Afraid you're going to make a fool of yourself on your first date with the new girl? Do something out of the ordinary that will make both of you laugh.

Leaders always have one thing on their side: courage. Sometimes you may have to go it alone, and that's when you need to face your fears straight on. That might make you uncomfortable, but you'll discover that the feeling doesn't last long and gives way to a tremendous sense of pride when you conquer it. Ultimately, people will respect you when you look fear in the eye and don't flinch—the bully who pushed you around after school, the beauty every guy's afraid to talk to, or all your classmates when you decide to run for class president even though you're shy. Best of all, you'll learn to respect yourself and to know that you can eclipse any fear that crosses your path.

My fear that cast the biggest shadow was stuttering. I had the tools to speak well, and there was no sign of the nasty stutter whenever I was with my family or friends. However, in a situation where I was less comfortable, such as talking in class or in front of people whom I didn't know (especially if I wanted to impress them), it would reappear and embarrass the heck out of me. It got so bad that my classmates took to calling me "Typewriter." Big J or Jako were nicknames I could live with, but Typewriter? It drove me nuts, but there was nothing I could do to get rid of it until I learned to face it down.

It's not an accident that I now run a business that forces me to speak in public many times a week. As long as I exercise my speech muscle as often as possible, the stuttering will stay in the closet! I have learned to use my fear as a continual positive source of energy and drive.

TRAINING TRIP-UP: *To Get Over the Intimidation Factor, Get Competitive!*

When I used to guard a huge dude in a basketball game—you know, like a six-foot-six, 230-pounder—I'd go right at him. I'd bump him off the block, stare at him without flinching, and show absolutely no pain no matter how hard we collided. It worked, because once he saw that I wasn't intimidated like most of his opponents, I had the mental edge and his game suffered. He might still make 15 points, but it wasn't going to be his usual 25!

I want you to carry the same attitude with you wherever you train. If you're by yourself, hit the weights without any fear. They will submit to your will, if your will is strong enough. Force them through another five reps, one more set! If you go to a gym, don't get intimated by the big fellow throwing around 110-pound dumbbells. Pick the right weight for you, and then train harder! Believe me, in the gym world, all it takes to get respect is training hard. And you'll always have that one covered! Even better, invite whatever fear you have into your workout so you can focus on getting over it. Fear is one training partner that you can obliterate every time!

Competition will always aid you in warding off fear. Occasionally, it's a great idea to seek it out before you're even ready, such as trying out for the school play even though you're the only one who was not a part of last year's play or joining an adult summer soccer league to raise your game. If you surround yourself with people who are more experienced or stronger than you, you're sure to join them sooner rather than later!

▪ Steamroll Over Any Setback, No Matter How Big ▪

There will be times, however, when a setback slams you to the turf. Maybe you weren't paying attention or were vulnerable at just that moment, but it can happen. It happened to me a number of years ago, when I made an appearance on Al Roker's weekend morning show on NBC. Before I went on, I was so relaxed that I felt like taking a nap in the waiting room. Without much warning, though, it was suddenly time to go on. A producer came to get me and took me out onto a small set where everybody was running around in a nervous frenzy. It was a live show, and I suddenly became as uptight as the atmosphere around me.

The interview started, and fear grabbed me by the throat. My brain-to-vocal-chords connection had blown a major fuse. The words I had planned to say wouldn't come out because my Stutter Monster was baaaack. I was again that ninth-grader stuttering away, humiliated in front of the class. This time, though, I was stumbling in front of a national TV audience! My five minutes with Al Roker seemed like five hours.

Here's the last part of the poem "Don't Quit":

DON'T QUIT POEM: *Failure Has a Flip Side!*

Success is failure turned inside out—
The silver tint of the clouds of doubt,
And you never can tell how close you are,
It may be near when it seems so far;
So stick to the fight when you're hardest hit—
It's when things seem worst that you must not quit.

Though I was upset with myself for a few hours, I quickly got some perspective from my wife, Tracey. I had lost a battle against the stuttering, despite having been winning the war for years. She advised me to reflect on my many victories—such as a talk I had given recently at the National Stutterer Convention, where my first sentence was shaky but I recovered quickly to deliver a great speech!—and not on my few losses. Just as when you get blindsided in a football game, the best response is always to jump right back up and act as though it didn't faze you, even if your knees wobble all the way back to the sideline! Accordingly, I was joking about that interview with friends later that same day. A few years later, after launching *Body by Jake* magazine, I made an appearance on the *Today* show with Al Roker, and it was a huge hit!

The truth is, everyone suffers setbacks—especially if you are expending a lot of effort chasing your dreams. I discovered that every single famous guy I trained had experienced failure before and knew that it would happen again. However, all of them had mastered the art of bouncing back more powerful than ever. There's one key reason: they never quit. Over the years I witnessed that process again and again, where these guys I looked up to would fail—in their business ventures and personal lives—but recover quickly to build greater successes.

Take the right tack, and a setback will be only a temporary slowdown. First, be flexible and have a backup plan. Failed your algebra test? Maybe it's time you asked for help from your neighbor the math whiz. Been rejected by your chosen girl for the prom? Have somebody else in mind who you're pretty sure will go with you. Act quickly without losing your cool, and these setbacks will barely register with you later on.

Second, the more serious the setback, the more you need your family, friends, and mentors to help. Look to them not just for support, but also to supply you with ideas about how to regroup. Demand honesty from these helpers so this setback becomes a learning experience that doesn't have to be repeated!

Third, write down what has happened. This helps you see the event clearly and forces you to come up with a solution. You may try this process in your mind, but only on paper can you plot out how to get beyond the setback.

Fourth, get ready to try again. If you're confident and know how you're going to go about it, success is around the corner!

DREAM EXTREME: *From Stuttering to Stand-up!*

Even with a pronounced fear of public speaking since childhood, I dreamed of being a stand-up comedian. Always the class clown in school and an aficionado of doing imitations, I relied upon humor to be accepted and overcome my insecurity about my stutter. While renewing my *Body by Jake* television series at a meeting of the National Association of Producers and Television Executives, I ran into the creator of *Evening at the Improv,* Budd Friedman. I told him I loved his show and would love to host it someday. I never mentioned doing a comic bit, because I didn't feel like getting my initiation into stand-up on a syndicated comedy show.

Much to my surprise, Budd called me the next week to invite me to not only host but also perform a stand-up routine with "four minutes of material." Have you heard the expression "Be careful what you wish for, you just might get it"? It was a huge risk—not for my business necessarily, but for my pride. All the questions that must occur to every comedian before he goes on were going through my head weeks in advance!

The night finally came. Backstage, I poked my head through the curtain and saw a bunch of hip, sophisticated people taking their seats. This could be Disasterville. I was sweating as if I'd been on the stair climber for half an hour. I certainly wasn't soothed by Garry Shandling, one of the top comics any-where, who walked up to me backstage and said, "You look pretty nervous, Jake."

"I am, Garry," I responded, hoping for some last-minute advice. "Don't worry, buddy. You're gonna bomb." He laughed, but I didn't. Next thing I knew a producer was tapping me on the back and telling me I was on. I grabbed the microphone, took a deep breath, and went out to kill or be killed—in comedian lingo.

I started with a story about being the world's only Jewish bodybuilder. They laughed. I told a bar mitzvah story. They laughed again. I told them that bodybuilders prefer making egg-white omelets to making whoopee. They laughed harder.

The red light came on, indicating that it was time for me to introduce the night's first comic. I ignored it and told another story. A dream had come true in a big way, and I wasn't about to go to sleep yet!

▪ Step Forward into the Leader Spot ▪

Once you deal with all the issues discussed in this chapter, you're ready to be a leader. Few guys want to assume the mantle, however, and are content to be a follower. They dress and talk the way everybody else does, find out what others are doing on the weekend before they make their plans, poll their peers before deciding what's and who's cool and what isn't.

When I was in high school, if you got on the bus wearing a funny-looking shirt, you'd hear more than your fair share of "you look stupid" comments. For most guys, that shirt would be off by lunchtime! I, though, always admired the fella who kept that shirt on and was his own man. It took guts to be different then, and it still does today.

I urge you to be different from your peers, whenever it feels right. *You* decide what's cool, who's worth being friends with, what class you're planning to take or sport you're going to go out for, instead of waiting to see which way the peer pendulum will swing. Just as you are the boss of the weights in your training room, be the boss among your own group of friends. Be the big guy in the room who, when everybody else is going left, says, "We're going right."

To get people to follow you, though, you have to carry yourself like a leader. That means: Develop your own style—the way you talk to people; your body language; how you dress. Treat everyone equally, and listen to all. Don't watch others to see what they're going to do next, but go your own way every time. Let your unique goals, such as training to become more muscular, inspire others.

Go first whenever you have the opportunity. Be the first one to write a paper on not just life during the French Revolution, but how theater may have affected life at the time; the first on your team to use plyometrics to improve your explosiveness; the first to befriend the new kid in school. That way you'll be taking the steps that will bring you the kind of future you prize, and in the process you will show your peers what leadership is all about.

I realized that going first into something was almost always a win-win situation, because I found more success when creating an idea where many others could share in that success. My subject was fitness, but I made it unique in my own way. Later I went on to become the first trainer to the stars, the first guy to bring fitness to TV, the first to start a major lacrosse league. Along the way, I helped a lot of people. Where will you go with your ideas?

YOU HOLD THE TICKETS TO A
GREAT FUTURE

Maybe they're not in your hands yet, but they're around somewhere—perhaps swept under a rug some time ago, or waiting to be created in your mind. I'm talking about *goals*. You've listened, looked in the mirror, learned to believe in yourself, tested your MQ, started training with me, and jumped some hurdles. Together, these experiences will help push you toward success, but if you truly want the successes that you've been dreaming about, you need to define your goals.

Leaving them undefined is like setting out in your V-12 to a foreign destination without looking at a map. You've heard what makes a great leader, except for this: A leader knows where he's headed. Now that you want to lead, it's essential to lay your goals out in front of you. Perhaps this is the first time you're determining goals for yourself. Your mom tells you that you should do this, your teacher tells you to do that, but now you're ready to spell out what exactly you want for yourself. Plus, you'll learn how to take it one day at a time, so that you won't get overwhelmed with the future.

What does "success" mean to you? Maybe it's muscles, grades, girls, sports, what college you get into, or girls (oops, I already said that). Actually, I deliberately repeated "girls" because that is what so often happens. You develop a one-track mind and think "girls, girls, girls" or "lacrosse, lacrosse, lacrosse." Instead, develop a many-track mind! Why not have it all?

Once you figure out the many types of successes that you want, I'll help you to prioritize them. Then it's up to you to go after those goals, hard!

▪ Ready, Get Set, Goal! ▪

You've arrived at the starting block ready to blast off, but which race are you in, and what goal are you after? If you don't know what you really want, then you're bound to wander around aimlessly—no matter how physically and mentally fit you are.

At Cortland State, I was in the best shape of my young life and willing to work really hard for what I believed in. Unfortunately, however, nothing on that campus—except for their dungeon of a weight room—represented a goal of mine.

My parents had grave doubts that bodybuilding in L.A. would lead to anything promising, but they also knew that it was far better to let me put all of my energy into chasing a dream than into sitting in college classes without a clue or a goal! I'll always be grateful for their faith in me, because while bodybuilding wasn't meant to be (for reasons I'll get into in the next chapter), L.A. was definitely the place for me. Also, my parents helped me make a tremendous discovery: Any goal, even if it doesn't fit you later on, is worth having, because it brings you closer to what you want from life.

If you feel like others are always making you do things you prefer not to do, or that bad things always seem to happen to you, then there's a good chance that you don't have a goal. Or if you blame interruptions for never getting enough done or you finish everything late because of some "excuse," you're probably without a goal, as well. It's easy to blame someone or something for not making the grade or the team, but the fault actually rests with you. Keep going without goals or focus, and you'll end up like me on that lacrosse field in mid-March—out in the cold, wondering how you got there in the first place.

Believe in your dreams and base your goals on them, and that destructive cycle is finally broken. Instantly, you will create and control your own destiny!

MUSCLE MAKER: *Put Yourself and Your Goals Into the Game!*

As you will find out, training helps you get to your goals if you invite those goals into your workout. As you try to push your muscles to the next stage during every workout—such as cranking out two more pull-ups than last time or adding ten more pounds on the squat—think about how you're going to do the same with your goal. "Lift this weight for another set, and master one more monologue later today." "Run another half mile, and read one more chapter in my astrophysics book."

Training injects a competitive spirit into the pursuit of your goals and helps you attain them in a shorter amount of time! Ever notice that you play harder in a competitive game than when you're just goofing around? That's because the goal becomes more compelling.

So, what do you have in mind? No, not a backstage pass to your favorite rap group in concert, but a serious goal that will move you forward. Choose a goal that you're willing to invest your time and energy in, day after day. At the same time, you'll waste less of your energy and creativity on things that have nothing to do with your goals.

To make your goal come alive, pursue it with passion. Whether you want to be an astronaut or an actor, I want your goal to excite you every day. Remind yourself of how incredible it will feel to be successful in that goal, and you'll work even harder to achieve it.

Additionally, be sure that your goal is for *you* and nobody else—not for your father, grandmother, or girlfriend. It will never work out as well unless it's your goal and your plan from the beginning. You won't get into great shape just because your mother thinks you are fat, or be accepted by a top law school because your uncle says it's the college that will make your future. Support of your goals from these loved ones is always welcome, and often crucial; you also want them to be proud of you when you achieve your goal, but you should want it for *you*. Great freedom and power will result.

REALITY CHECK: *I'm Not My Father, and That's Okay*

Fathers always want their sons to do well, especially if they suspect that Junior doesn't have any goals. In my father's eyes, chasing my bodybuilding dreams out in L.A. was akin to having no goal at all. Consequently, he tried to turn me into a salesman like he was. Living nearby, he sold advertising for his own magazine and did well for himself. He figured I was due for a real job, so he asked that I give ad sales a shot.

My father set up a sales call for me to go on to see one of his clients, a florist. I wasn't aware of it then, but he actually promised the florist a free ad if he would play along by making it tough for me to get a "sale." My father knew that sales wasn't my first love but calculated that if the florist played hard to get, my competitive juices would kick in and winning him over would be as much fun as becoming Mr. America.

For him, I tried—even wore a suit and tie. I arrived at the florist's shop with my dad's magazine under my arm and asked to meet the owner. He came out, and I said, "Hi, I'm Jake Steinfeld. I would like to offer you the inside front cover for $850."

He looked at the magazine for a second and said, "No thanks."

Relieved, I blurted out, "Okay, thanks!" Then I turned and walked out before the astonished florist could say a word.

My father was waiting at his office smiling, since he figured his little scheme had worked like a charm.

"So, how'd it go?" he asked.

"The guy at the florist shop said no," I said, shrugging my shoulders.

"Of course he said no! I asked him to give you a hard time, but to take the ad anyway. I was testing you. You doofus!" he shot back.

After his anger quickly wore off, however, he recognized that I simply was not committed to being an ad salesman. He realized that was *his* dream for me, instead of my own. I wanted to find my own way, and now he understood that.

▪ Develop Your Dreams into Goals ▪

Now that you have some good ideas about what you want, you're ready to turn them into specific and concrete goals. Instead of opting for a vague goal like losing weight or making the team, tell yourself you're going to lose fifteen pounds and become the starting forward! Perhaps you dream of getting into the college of your choice or becoming a famous photographer; so concentrate on earning straight A's this next semester, or putting on an exhibit in your hometown.

When defining your goals, don't look too far ahead into the future. Start relatively small, by laying out goals that you can visualize meeting in the coming days, weeks, and months—goals that jack you up the moment you wake up in the morning! The successful Hollywood people whom I trained never had just one large goal way off in the distance; instead, they had several smaller goals that served as stepping stones to greater goals.

Therefore, while I encourage you to reach for more than you think you can accomplish, you should set goals that are manageable in the short term in order for the long-term goals to remain in range! For example, chalk up some wins each day. Even if they are small things—such as contributing in class, eating a healthy lunch, chatting with your dream girl after school, having a great workout—they add up over time into something big! Just as doing your homework every day makes it a lot easier to pass that test down the line, small victories make it more probable that you will meet your goal (which will be more fun than taking that test!). Each day your confidence grows as you keep churning on that path to your goals. I've witnessed it countless times: success breeds greater success!

POWER HABIT: *Set Goals and Stick to Them*

Find a quiet place to get comfortable, where you won't get interrupted and where your mind is free of all the clutter. Enter your imaginary world, where you're going to create some goals.

1. Ask yourself what you want: turn your focus toward the goals you want to pursue now and in the future. What will make you feel fulfilled *and* improve the environment around you? What makes you happy *and* taps your potential to the fullest extent? Typically, they go hand-in-hand, since many people are happiest when using their talents as much as possible. What can you envision that will excite you today, tomorrow, and the next day? How about a year or five years from now?

2. Prioritize the goals: whether you came up with a list of two or twelve, weigh the value that each of them holds for you. You have only so much time and energy to spend, so before you shoot for the moon, make sure

your top goals can be attended to every day. Otherwise, spreading yourself too thin may jeopardize all of your goals.

3. Map out the path: how do you think you're going to arrive at your goal? Think about the steps and minigoals that will move you closer to the big goal.

4. Visualize the pursuit: any goal worth its salt requires sacrifices and changes in your life. Imagine how each day will be different with this goal in your life. If going after it in your mind creates any doubts that this goal is worth it, then it most likely isn't. However, if you can honestly say to yourself, "I want this, no matter what it takes," then it's the perfect goal for you!

5. Put it on paper: whether you decide to put it down in words or in a drawing, your goal and its map need to be somewhere else besides in your mind. The very act of creating it in your notebook, computer, or personal journal brings it to life. After you write down all your goals, say them out loud to reinforce the fact that these goals are now real and just waiting to be met.

6. Soak in the good feeling: accomplishing your goal will bring you great satisfaction and pride. Imagine yourself at various points in the future getting near or meeting each goal, and how tremendous it feels to be using all your talents and resources for these goals. Dig up this feeling any time you need a boost.

7. A day at a time: don't feel overwhelmed by the future or intimidated by these goals, no matter how grand they are. Instead, every night, think of what you can do the next day that will help you to reach your goals, and put it down on your "Power List" (see Chapter 3) for tomorrow.

8. Sunday Night Live!: before I had any goals as a teenager, I'd get sick to my stomach on Sunday night thinking of the upcoming school week. The Sunday night strategy, however, will replace that dread with excitement. First, look back on the past week and run through the seven steps above. Second, make adjustments to your goals, such as expanding your vision to include related goals or adding something altogether new. Third, set a date on the calendar for certain accomplishments. Keep it realistic and accomplishable!

You're young with many decisions ahead of you—so some of these goals may change quite a bit over the years. Don't let that fact, however, prevent you from setting and pursuing your goals, because the worst that can happen to you in pursuing a goal is twenty times better than the best that you can do with no goal at all. Why? Because once you begin to chase goals, you create momentum in your life that simply makes good things happen, from goal capturing to creating other goals, to just being in a good mood!

▪ Work and Patience Lead to a Big Payoff ▪

Let's face it, few people are really willing to work hard for their goals. They expect success overnight—a few hours spent on an essay is good enough to earn an A; one phone call to that great girl will result in a date; a week of good practices assures starting the next game—but it doesn't work that way. *You're* not going to make that mistake, because you know it's going to take sweat and guts to make your goals come out like you have envisioned . . . just as you know that it might take a month or two of working out to see the muscle you want.

The bonus is that your effort becomes enjoyable, regardless of your goal, which, in turn, aids your pursuit of that goal. You'll see the effort begin to pay off: the extra hours you devote to crafting a really good paper; the cool conversations you get into with the dream girl, which make a date a sure thing; the intense contribution you give your team during every minute of every practice to ensure you a starter slot. You'll see the same pattern in your workouts: the more you give, the greater will be your enjoyment level, as well as your results.

That's not to say that you won't get sidetracked once in a while. Sitting down at night to do your homework, for example, might sometimes be the last thing you have in mind—it certainly was for me! Often, every half hour or less, you take one undeserved break after the next: flip on the TV, place a call to a friend, listen to a CD, go make a snack for yourself. Consequently, it takes you hours longer to finish your homework, or you don't finish it at all!

Instead, I urge you to focus the same way you do with your workout. Begin your homework in a positive frame of mind and be completely ready to go—make sure you've already used the facilities, informed your family that you're not to be disturbed, had your glass of water, gotten rid of the distractions, closed the door, and are stationed at your desk with all your materials. Then commit to an hour of straight work, just like the workout. Soon you'll get into it, as time flies and the work gets done. Once again, as in the workout, efficiency is a very useful skill to have on your side. Take a small break after an hour to refresh yourself, and then get back on that horse. Follow this routine, and you'll finish your homework at a more reasonable hour and have time to spare for other interests.

You can become sidetracked with any other goal, as well, so keep your eyes on the prize. Whenever you need an extra push, remind yourself of the rewards and benefits that will come your way after reaching your goals.

■ The Biggest of Them All: Your Ultimate Goal ■

Getting into great physical shape can start you on your journey and help you to keep moving forward, but what are you moving toward? While training some of the most successful people in show business, I realized that, for them, training to reach body perfection was certainly not the big goal. It made them feel and look great, but the most important thing it accomplished was to enable them to advance to the next level—in their careers, relationships, finances, education, you name it. On top of their many goals, however, the great motivator for them was the *ultimate goal*—whether it was fame, critical acclaim, or fabulous wealth.

All your other goals should revolve around this ultimate goal, which serves as the sun in your personal universe. Like the pilot who constantly adjusts his course by checking his instruments, you must determine whether you are on course by repeatedly checking whether your actions are in alignment with your ultimate goal.

Unlike lesser goals, your ultimate goal concerns much more than your present interests and hopes. Instead, it's all about the future. Perhaps your ultimate goal will take you three years or thirty years to reach—that depends on you and the goal you choose. Whatever it is, your ultimate goal should give you a picture for your mind to focus on each day.

Maybe your ultimate goal right now is finding the perfect girl. That will lead you directly to related goals like gaining more muscle, speaking better, and exuding more confidence. Develop those related goals first, and your chances at getting the biggie—the girl—are much better. That's how it works: Whatever you do during your day, you can use the image of this girl to motivate you further.

As a teenage guy, I longed to become Mr. America. That was my ultimate goal. That meant all my smaller goals fell into line with the big one, such as never missing a workout and giving every ounce of energy I had to my training. Or giving up all the junk food for healthy, muscle-building food. Having that ultimate prize waiting for me prevented me from wandering off course.

And while the ultimate goal usually takes most guys to college, it persuaded me to leave college and live in L.A.!

Pretty quickly, though, that Mr. America prize didn't seem like enough for me. Soon after arriving in L.A., I replaced it with my decision to become an entrepreneur in the health and fitness field. My first step toward that goal was to become a personal trainer, then I decided to augment that by creating some fitness books and videos. My ultimate goal remained larger than those accomplishments, though, so I kept driving forward. Inspired by what I had seen Ted Turner, the cable TV guru, create when I was doing my fitness tips for CNN, I wanted, next, to have my own multifaceted multimedia company. Ultimately, I made Body by Jake a household brand name and created my own twenty-four-hour cable network centered on health and fitness called FiT TV.

As soon as you realize that your ultimate goal is not ultimate enough, you put something bigger in its place. When you choose a career path, for instance, you'll notice that there are many different ways to go—although you will only become aware of that fact once you've begun to make headway on a goal. I hoped to be a bodybuilder and pursued that intensely for years, but soon I recognized that the fitness world had bigger things in store for me than simply bodybuilding.

Perhaps you love biology and your ultimate goal is to become a doctor, but that goal ends up being replaced by your desire to be a veterinarian. Or your passion is playing sports and your ultimate goal is gaining an athletic scholarship to a university, where your ultimate goal changes into something completely unrelated to sports. As your ultimate goal changes, so do all the goals underneath it. What remains fixed is your desire to keep climbing that mountain!

▪ Your First Thought? "I Can Do This" ▪

"I will build the body I want for myself." "I will get the girl I'm dreaming about." "I will get into the college of my choice." Put these thoughts front and center in your mind, and tend to them every day, then these ambitions will take shape.

You don't learn this in school, but success is a decision you make. You're the only guy who will decide whether or not you will relentlessly pursue success, and your decisions along the way will determine how successful you become. Every goal you make, every action you take, begins with a decision.

You decide what time you're going to get up in the morning—whether to make it to school on time, or to get up even earlier to get in a workout and breakfast. You decide how you're going to participate in class—only if you're forced, or frequently and intelligently. It goes on throughout the day. You decide if you're going to chat with the dream girl. You decide how hard you're going to work in sport practice or some other extracurricular activity. You decide who you're going to hang out with after school. You decide how hard you're going to hit the books that night.

The quality of these decisions predicts the level of success you'll have that day. Every day, every week, for the rest of your life depends on these kinds of decisions, not on your wishes—because there's a huge difference between a decision and a wish. A wish means that you hope something good happens for you, but you remain stationary, not taking any action. A decision, meanwhile, is all about action. It propels you forward toward all those goals.

POWER HABIT: *Decide to Decide!*

As you grow older and your goals grow in size, your decisions become only more serious. If you make one good, smart decision after another, you'll wind up exactly where you want to be. Here's a rundown of the factors you should consider before making each decision:

1. Stack it up against your ultimate goal: how does your decision fit in with your short-term and long-term goals? Does it put you closer or farther away? Or have no effect at all?

2. Ponder the positive and the negative: most likely, it will have an impact. Play it out carefully in your mind, then write down the positives and negatives in different columns. If the negative side fills up faster than the positive side, bail. If it's still unclear, then the risk is up to you!

3. Trust your gut: if it remains unclear what to do, go with your instincts. Do what you heart tells you, then even if it doesn't work out, at least you don't beat yourself up about it.

4. Make the decision: whatever you do, decide now. Don't leave it behind, telling yourself you'll come back and decide later. You need to keep moving!

When I look at my pals Steven Spielberg and Harrison Ford, I recognize the huge hurdles they flew over to get to where they are now. Wiels came from a troubled family and yet *decided* to rise above his circumstances to pursue his dreams of making films. Harrison flunked out of college and *decided* that he could be a successful actor. Me? Well, you know my story pretty well by now! I was a fat kid with a stutter who *decided* I could be a highly successful entrepreneur.

You're no different. In weight lifting, it's not merely the poundage you hoist, but the number of reps you decide to do that builds the muscle you want. In getting to your goals, the more decisions you make, the stronger your decision-making powers become. You will, however, make some doozies along the way, too. Why? Because nobody can predict the future. A great decision one day could be a stinker the next. As a result, it's crucial that you understand the potential risks and rewards.

In getting to your ultimate goal, sometimes the grueling step-by-step approach won't cut it. If you've either had an unexpected success or picked up momentum, you're ready to seize the opportunities that exist. If you've simply stalled out, it may be time to take a risk. Regardless of whether you view it as an opportunity or a risk, take it, because you're hungry to succeed and not scared to fail. In fact, if you *don't* fail, then you're not pushing yourself hard enough!

Taking risks is the way to grow, but don't take them if they might ruin your reputation or ground your flight to the ultimate goal. Instead, each risk must qualify as a risk you're more than willing to take. First, you should know exactly what you want to accomplish. Second, you must prepare for some bad consequences as well as good ones, because by their very nature, many risks fail. So have a plan of action ready. Third, never take a risk for your ego alone. Finally, take your risk with confidence and enjoy the experience!

DREAM EXTREME: *Blowing All My Savings on a Car?*

Okay, it was a black Mercedes 380SL, not just any old car. With all my V-12 talk, you're hardly surprised! However, it was a big risk back then. I had saved $10,000 from my personal training business and was prepared to put a down payment on a condominium. It was the smart, sensible thing to do rather than keep throwing money down the drain with my monthly rent checks. Then it hit me. I said to myself, "Forget the boring condo, I'm going to buy a Mercedes-Benz."

I withdrew $9,400 from my bank account and plunked it down on the Merc. Confident that it was the right move? I'm afraid not. In fact, those monthly car payments were higher than my rent. But it was a calculated gamble that could put my career in the fast lane! I was left with only $600 in the bank, which put considerable pressure on me to be successful very quickly. It was a challenge that I was happy to accept. Anyway, I was prepared to sleep in my car before giving it away!

Note that I didn't get this car just to look cool (although that didn't hurt!). I did it to boost my business. Hollywood runs on image, so when clients and potential clients saw me in this sweet Merc, I was no longer the gym instructor. I was now the successful personal trainer and businessman. From then on, every article written about me always mentioned this line: "Jake pulls up to his celebrity client's home in his black Mercedes-Benz. . . ."

Sometimes you have to play the game if you want to score. I landed even bigger clients, then journeyed into the book publishing world shortly afterward. I owed part of my newfound success to the little Merc that still remains parked in my garage today.

▪ Meeting Big Goals and Making Big Changes ▪

Your goals will usher in some changes in your life. Then once you meet some of these goals, even more radical changes will occur. Change, however, isn't a walk in the park—as you already know from your teenage life. Whether it was your first day of high school or the first time you kissed a girl, change can be terrifying or tremendous. Change is all about how you respond.

Often, change takes you out of your comfort zone, and that's when fear and uncertainty can strike. If the change encompasses something that you have no control over, such as your parents getting divorced, it can be a vicious blow. Or it could be something you had a lot to do with, such as losing your summer job or a bad breakup with your girlfriend. To cope successfully with change, expect some rocky times; feelings of loneliness, self-doubt, and despair are common whenever you're jolted from your comfort zone.

Many people, however, run right back into their comfort zone because they're unable to handle the emotional roller coaster of change. It's what keeps many stuck in place and unable to go after what they want. They're unwilling to give up what is familiar, even if they are unhappy, because they're afraid to face the unknown.

I urge you to go boldly where you haven't gone before! Many changes, in fact, are positive ones if you choose to look at them that way, especially if they occur as a result of your goals. Take your goal of getting into great physical shape as an example. Doing these four workouts a week might force you to miss watching your favorite TV show or joining your pals at the mall. Eating healthy means the chicken breast sandwich rather than a cheeseburger. These represent changes that yank you out of your comfort zone, but ones that you and your goal are better off with.

STUMBLING . . . TO SUCCESS: *From Womba to Big Brother Jake*

Part of me always itches to try something different. One day when I was training at my gym, an actor-friend of mine gave me the opportunity to have a role in an upcoming film. My personal training business was barely off the ground, so it sounded cool to me!

That actor was Tommy Chong, of the Cheech and Chong comedy duo. Although he'd do the entertaining on the big screen, during our workouts he preferred to laugh at my stories and jokes, especially the tales that surrounded my gig playing the Incredible Hulk on the Universal Studios Tour. Doused in green paint, I'd supply comic relief to the audience. It wasn't Best Actor material, but Tommy thought it would be perfect for the sequel to their hit *Up in Smoke.*

So as not to get into a trademark battle with those who owned the real Hulk name, my character's name was changed to Womba and the color to red. Tommy brought the script to the gym for me to read, and I was stunned. This bumbling red superhero had a costarring role, a huge part for a guy who had never even been on a movie set. It was a hilarious part, with Womba walking through the wrong walls and always rescuing the wrong people.

I was geared up for some changes. But when the producer told my parents that I "was going to be a big star," it looked like I'd hit the jackpot! I called all my friends back in Long Island to inform them a star was born. I had my own trailer on the set with all the food I could eat. I was one lucky guy.

Day three, however, my luck changed in an instant. The line producer told me the studio executives loved my work, but that they had a problem: "a 245-pound guy painted red dominates every scene in the movie and that is not the star they're paying for. They're paying for Cheech and Chong." Just like that, I was cut from the movie.

For a while after that, I couldn't get my mind's eye off the door that was closing rather than focusing on what was opening up. This change was really out of my hands, yet I couldn't help feeling sorry for myself. Soon, though, I realized that it opened many other doors. I no longer wanted to have some producer decide my fate. It gave me the incentive to build my business in my "bread-and-butter" field of fitness and create my own luck.

Years afterward, when my business was going strong, I decided to write my own script rather than get written out of one! I created a sitcom where I'd play the central character, a big brother who was in charge of the household. Most of the network executives wanted to change the concept to a story in which I played either a personal trainer or a bodyguard. They just didn't believe in my idea. Finally, someone did: Tim Robertson, president of the Family Channel. The TV show *Big Brother Jake* went on to become a big hit on the Family Channel.

The older guy who tells you that "high school is the best time of your life"—the "glory days"—is someone afraid of change. He never let go in order to move onward and upward. I certainly want your high school experience to be a great one, and that's partly what motivated me to write this book. However, overall I'm most interested in helping you create a great *life*. To do that, continue to move forward no matter what change occurs for you. If you hit a snag, hang in there; your confidence and energy will return in no time!

Life is a nonstop adventure if you live it that way, and high school is only the beginning. Master the ability to deal with change, and you'll be able to face any challenge without blinking!

nine

You've learned how to develop your goals, from building muscle to building your future. To maximize the potential of these goals, however, you can't do it all on your own. You need someone or something that will help push you toward your goals and keep you on track whenever you veer off course. Go-To People and good nutrition make up that support staff.

Do you have someone to go to when the going gets tough? If you do, that someone is your Go-To Person. If you don't, it's time to search him or her out. A Go-To Person knows how to boost your confidence, yet still give you a kick in the buttissimo, depending on what you need at that moment! Their support of you is so strong that often they want your dreams to come true as badly as you do. My ultimate Go-To Person was my grandma Myra Duberstein, who believed in me no matter what happened.

Getting the muscled physique you prize takes a different kind of support, but one just as constant: solid nutrition. After training so hard with those weights, you want to capitalize on your gains by eating to jack up the muscle and keep the fat down. Just as I gave you the tools to work your muscles in the best way possible, now I hand you the tools to develop an eating plan that you trust and will use every week. (Don't worry, you get one day per week to eat anything you want.) Plus, you'll see that you don't have to tame your desire for great taste and variety!

Be aware that your support system doesn't exist on its own. First, you still have to seek out the people and the eating plan that works for you. Second, to improve the level of effectiveness for you, remain faithful to these people and your muscle diet. The more you do that, the greater your successes will be.

On the flip side, there are many potentially damaging people who block the way to your goals. Meanwhile, many "performance-enhancing" drugs might appear to aid your trip down the path to your goal of more muscle, but turn out to be just as damaging. I'm going to show you that your *natural* support system is all you need!

▪ Go Farther with Your Go-To Person ▪

Undoubtedly, you've heard of the "Go-To Guy" on each sports team. He's the player who, when the chips are down, will deliver whatever his team needs to win the game. Shaquille O'Neal, center for the Los Angeles Lakers basketball team, is an example. Even though he's complemented by the outstanding player Kobe Bryant, there's no doubt that he's the guy his teammates can always rely on, game in and game out.

A Go-To Person does the same for you—someone who is always there for you, who believes in you and your dreams, and who is willing to help you out in any way possible. On the way to your ultimate goal, you will face challenging times. These can hamper your progress and erode your confidence, but your Go-To Person will keep you focused and inspired to reach your goals, which will make all the difference. Most of all, in a world where many tend toward negativity, your Go-To remains positive that you can do it at all times!

Your family is the most natural source for Go-To's: one or both of your parents whom you can always depend on, or maybe an older brother or sister. Be aware that not everyone is so lucky. Some guys have their entire clan pulling for them—attending every game, aware of every college they applied to, slapping 'em on the back at every family picnic—but maybe you don't have it so easy. Your older brother shouts out, "Dork is in the house," every time you crack a book, while your father hasn't made it to one of your games since T-ball.

Parents who put their own wishes for you to the side and give you their full support to pursue what you want are rare. If that doesn't describe your parents, be understanding. They have so much emotionally invested in you that they worry if you try anything risky or go outside a prescribed path. Perhaps they don't understand your dream or think it worthy of your time. Remember: They feel responsible not only for your happiness and security, but also for your future.

My parents were always loving and supportive, yet they had very different ideas about my future than I did. They were pleased to see my enthusiasm for fitness, but frankly didn't see how that would pay the bills one day! For a nice boy from Baldwin, New York, a doctor or lawyer was the ticket. A body-builder? That was a one-way trip to nowhere.

Fortunately, when it comes to the Go-To category, all you need is *one* person. Grandma Duberstein was such an all-encompassing Go-To Person that I really didn't need another until later in my life, after she passed away. Even if you live in an unsupportive environment, see if you have one family member who will listen to you and offer guidance at any hour; otherwise, maybe you have a teacher, coach, or older student who wants to serve as your mentor.

Once you know who your Go-To Person is, be aware that it's not a one-way street: Your commitment to him or her is just as important as your Go-To Person is to you. If you want that person's advice, you must listen. Equally, if you want your Go-To Person's time whenever you have a need, then you must invest your time into the relationship.

The return on this investment is sky-high, because you develop a more meaningful relationship for both of you, as well as set yourself up for a more rewarding future. The more involved your Go-To is with your future, the more motivated and unafraid you will be in going after it. No matter what you do or where you go, in all cases, from your darkest moments to your shining successes, you will always have that Go-To Person right behind you.

GO-AWAY PEOPLE

Always outnumbering your Go-To crew are those whom I call the Go-Away People. Not only do they not support you and your dreams, but they may, in fact, try to hold you back from achieving them because of jealousy, selfishness, or disrespect. Perhaps they constantly doubt you and put you down. Maybe, instead, they hardly involve themselves with you at all and simply exist as a negative presence.

When facing a challenge—such as a tough obstacle, a constant fear, or a recent failure—the last thing you need is someone who offers no hope or guidance. People like this are usually unhappy for their own reasons and are simply bringing it to your doorstep, but I ask you not to let them inside. Help them out if you can, then move on. Poisonous people get their fangs in you and kill your goals dead in their tracks. This poison can be released by the guys you pal around with. It may seem cool to join them in being cynical and sarcastic, but that attitude can infect you after a while. They may not want to see you get ahead or change in any way, because they haven't.

You need to either cut these people out of your life or distance yourself from them if you truly want to achieve your goals. If you're unsure of who deserves the ax, all you have to do is ask the following three questions:

1. Do they make you better or do they drag you down?

2. Do they care about your goals or could they not care less about your progress?

3. Are their own lives on an upward spiral, or are they stuck or in a tailspin?

▪ Go-To Grams ▪

The one person who is most responsible for where I am today is Grandma Duberstein. All throughout my childhood and teenage years, she invested huge amounts of time—and probably money—in preparing me for success. Actually, I thought she was loaded—she seemed to know everybody in New York City. She managed the Manhattan Beach Hotel in Manhattan, where many famous people stayed. From singers to basketball stars, she befriended them all. I loved helping her out there, checking coats and earning tips.

Go-To Grams knew my life was limited out in Long Island, so she did whatever she could to show me the world. It became her mission. Whatever great event was going on in the city, she would manage to swing a pair of tickets through her hotel contacts or through an aquaintance guarding the back entrance! From sports (U.S. Open tennis matches, Mets games, ski resorts in upstate New York, boxing matches) to culture (museum special exhibits, plays, music concerts, movies) I got to experience it, with my horizon broadening all the while.

She didn't take me to sit in the cheap seats, however. If Grandma noticed a famous athlete or movie star in the crowd, she'd tug me along to introduce herself and me to them as if we were celebrities, too. I still have all those childhood photos with my sports heroes and Hollywood stars, as well as their autographs. Did we ever get turned down? Only once. When I was eight years old, she asked Mets stars Tom Seaver and Jerry Grote to sign my baseball glove. Seaver smartly obliged, but Grote ignored us. She gave him a few choice words, then turned to me and said, "When you're famous, don't ever be like that man."

I smiled and nodded, but inwardly I found it unlikely that I'd ever be a name anyone would know. Go-To Grams's belief in me was so powerful, though, that she knew I was headed toward great things. After years of being around her motivating and positive presence, my own belief in my abilities got stronger. I began to understand that something special waited for me out there, as long as I was willing to do the work.

When I left college to become a bodybuilder, almost everyone second-guessed me—except for her. After seeing my commitment to building the best body I could, she was confident it would lead to grander things beyond a bronze trophy. When I competed in the Mr. Southern California contest, she flew out to support me even though she was very sick. I wanted to win for her, but I came in second.

In typical Grandma Duberstein fashion, she said, "Don't worry about it; you will win the next one."

She never got to see me try. At her funeral, I stood next to her casket and felt my knees shake. I was only twenty years old, and the most important person in my life was gone. She was barely five feet, four inches long in that coffin, but she was much bigger than that: She was bigger than *life*. Today, her spirit remains by my side. Anytime I catch myself feeling negative or taking a defeatist attitude, I imagine her encouraging voice and snap out of it.

POWER HABIT: *Getting Your Go-To*

Talking about Go-To People does nothing for you if you can't find one! Don't forget to look right in front of your eyes; you might actually spot one there! Follow these four easy steps to find the perfect Go-To for you:

1. Show total commitment to your dream: to attract the right Go-To Person, just let your energy and dedication to whatever goals you have show. Anybody, whether or not that person is a potential Go-To, will find this irresistible.

2. Find a role model: who do you look up to? Who is already where you want to be? Go to this person and ask for advice and help. If the response is enthusiastic, then you may have a Go-To!

3. Look for tough love: you want somebody in your corner who will always look out for you, but that doesn't mean he or she should support every move you make. On the contrary, when the situation calls for it and you need it, a great Go-To challenges you as well as points you in another direction.

4. Pick a positive partner: choose a friend who is going in the same direction as you and become a tag team. He or she will have different goals but should share your intense desire to get better every day. Compare notes, help each other, work out together—rise together!

▪ Your Go-To Leads to Your Ultimate Goal ▪

A Go-To Person not only has your back, but often can give you a little nudge whenever you appear to wander away from your ultimate goal. You, the student, need a teacher, and you, the athlete, need a coach to get the most of your scholastic and athletic abilities; the same is true for you, the young man with big plans. Perhaps you think you don't need any assistance in remaining focused on your goals, but it never hurts to have someone to steady you when you stumble, and offer a second opinion when you're uncertain.

For example, it's essential that your Go-To supports your training plan. Sticking to the four workouts per week and a good diet takes discipline and dedication, every day. You're human, so there will be days when you won't feel the urge to train or the desire to eat intelligently. Next thing you know, you've skipped your workout for a McDonald's run. How can you get back on track? Your Go-To can remind you of your commitment to training and the rewards, and possibly provide you with the healthy food you need to build your body. Maybe your Go-To Person will join you in both efforts.

MUSCLE MAKER: *Go-To Exercises*

Just as a Go-To Person can get you out of any jam, a few Go-To Exercises can work your muscles no matter where you are . . . at your Aunt Helen's place, where you're bored stiff; in front of the TV when you're watching a game; or as a walk down the block to pick up a magazine. It may not be your day to train, but getting in a small workout can release tension and boost your mood, plus do your muscles some good. Try these few Go-To's:

1. Hustle: one fun practice is simply to sprint, rather than walk, when you are going from A to B. Next time you run an errand or are walking over to see a friend, sprint the whole way to build some more explosive power. You'll see the carryover when you step on the athletic field, and plus you might well get more things done during your day!

2. Push-up: the ultimate upper-body exercise that you can do anywhere, any way. Hands in close for triceps, out wide for chest; elevate your feet to add difficulty, and do them on your knees when you get tired. The next time you plunk down to watch a game, bang out forty during commercials.

3. Walking lunge: it might look funny to walk across your house or around your backyard this way, but your thigh muscles will thank you. With an erect torso, take a large step forward and land softly. Drop your working leg until your thigh is parallel to the ground. Do not let the knee joint move past your toe. Work at a moderate pace: two seconds up, two seconds down. Start out with one set of ten reps on each side, working up to more sets as you advance.

4. Crunch: did you know that your stomach muscles recover more quickly than any of your other muscles? That means even if you trained them yesterday, you can still do a couple more sets as a homework break. Put a few more ribs in that washboard!

My Go-To Grams adopted my dream of bodybuilding as if it were her own. If she could have lifted weights right beside me, she would have. She took me to my first competitions in and around New York, and even helped douse me in tanning oil so my muscles would stand out under the lights. In my initial competition, I finished fifth out of thirty-five guys and was psyched. I told her, "I'm going to be Mr. America."

"You already are Mr. America," she replied. That's the way she always was with me, pumping my mind up, while I pumped up my muscles. Whenever we went out to a restaurant, she made it a point to choose a place where I could fill up on chicken breasts and good veggies. She understood every step toward my goal as much as I did.

Since she was two generations older than I was, however, my grandma knew she couldn't be my Go-To Person forever. One of the most valuable lessons she taught me was how to build and maintain relationships that were mutually supportive, and she encouraged me to find other people who would notice my potential and push me closer to my goals. Meanwhile, she taught me to give back whatever I could to these important people, and always to show tremendous loyalty to them.

She taught me well—she passed me on to a succession of Go-To People who helped me move up the mountain higher than I could ever have made it on my own. At the gym, I enthusiastically spotted professional bodybuilders, who then gave me many great tips on training and the bodybuilding business— eventually helping me to decide that it wasn't the right kind of business for me. When I began training members of the powerful Hollywood community, I did my best to make exercise productive *and* fun for them, and they, in turn, responded to me incredibly well and appreciated my dedication to getting them into great shape, and many became my new Go-To's.

STUMBLING . . . TO SUCCESS:
From Slasher Flicks to Serious Business

One of my first film roles was the distinguished one of the crazed killer in a horror film called *Home Sweet Home.* In my big scene, I murdered an entire family during their Thanksgiving Day dinner! Needless to say, these kinds of acting choices weren't going to lead to much, plus it was ruining my wardrobe—it took me weeks to get the blood (cherry syrup) out of my clothes!

As I delved further into the entertainment business and beyond, my Go-To People's advice made all the difference. Steven "Wiels" Spielberg, for instance, guided me toward the right choices in the extremely competitive environments of acting, TV programming, and eventually my own multimedia company.

A few years after getting to know Wiels, I was offered a role as costar in a new crime-fighter TV series. The other costar was a big, funny actor who mostly played himself in a cartoonish way that young people liked. The proposition was very tempting—good money and more exposure for the Body by Jake brand—but I was still unsure. I went to Wiels, who took about a half second to respond.

"Stop! I've got nothing against your costar. He's a nice guy, but do you really want to play second banana to a second banana? Forget about the TV exposure for a minute and think about the business you are trying to build. How would this impact your brand as a serious businessman?" he asked.

There it was; the answer that I needed to hear. I turned down the offer. It might have been fun and provided some excellent money, but by accepting the role, I risked being typecast and shrinking my future options. Wiels came through for me in a big way, and I only hope I can return the favor to him someday.

In a way, since I never finished college, my network of Go-To People became my college. The only difference was that I went to school in sweatpants, I called my professors by nicknames, and the student-to-teacher ratio was one to one! I didn't expect them to want to teach me all the time, however, as I was just as willing to help them in their challenges as well. In fact, I've served as a Go-To Person for many of these friends over the years.

I want you also to create your own network of Go-To's. It may take years, but you will never regret your investment into this never-ending source of support. Trust is the biggest part of your relationship to each Go-To Person you find. If people sense that the only reason you want a relationship with them is to further your own goals, trust will never develop. Instead, you must be willing to lend a hand if you expect others to do the same for you. Perhaps that means doing chores around the house for your Go-To Mom or Dad without being asked, or making sure your Go-To Coach is okay following the death of his relative. Continue to show your gratitude for their help in your actions and words, and your relationship will only grow in strength.

Eventually, you will become a Go-To Person yourself—first for your friends and younger siblings, if you have any, and then for your Go-To's themselves. After all, it's part of being the leader you want to be. Your mom gives you the responsibility of taking care of your younger sisters while she's away; your teacher appoints you to head the class project; your coach depends on you to pump up your teammates in the locker room.

Once people start to recognize your Go-To abilities and leadership skills, your Go-To Network is going to explode! The connections you need to make and the places you want to go will actually start coming to you, rather than you always chasing them down. I owe my business as a fitness motivator to word of mouth: one person recommended me to another person, and so on. The same will happen with your goal.

▪ Mentor Your Muscles with Great Food ▪

Just as you shouldn't choose those who are bad for you to be your Go-To People, you can't expect to have a superior performance if you are fueling yourself with nutritionally inferior food. Unfortunately, this truth escapes many hard-training guys—including some great athletes. The fact is that healthy eating can maximize your gains. Just as Go-To People bring out the best in you in your goal pursuit, a solid diet ensures that your muscles will receive the nutrients needed to grow maximally.

You know the old adage "You are what you eat"? I used to be a donut-and-Twinkie guy before I started training at age fourteen, and guess what I looked like! Yep, a glazed Twinkie! So if you're out there eating potato chips twenty-four/seven, you probably also prefer swimming with a T-shirt on to hide that Pringles label imprinted on your chest. Worse, eating that way doesn't give you the energy and stamina needed to make it a successful day, especially if you work out or play a sport.

Like many bad habits, this starts at home. While you're not helped by the nutritionally bankrupt meals typically served at your school, or by your friends' tendency to hit the drive-thru more than the weights, eating junk is a habit usually handed down from your parents. (If they eat healthfully, on the other hand, count yourself lucky.) Loaded with sugar, salt, and fat, these foods—like sugary cereals, white bread, butter, fatty meats, deep-fried vegetables, potato chips, "cheese puffs," sodas, ice cream, and cake—have little to offer except temporary pleasure and long-term chub. Plus, all the good you did for yourself during your workout is undone in fifteen minutes of shoveling garbage down your throat afterward!

Don't blame your parents for serving you this food, however, because they probably don't know any other way to shop for groceries or cook dinner. It simply means that they don't know it's possible to eat tasty and interesting fare that is also energizing and healthy. Now that *you* do, I'm challenging you to change your eating habits first, then perhaps they will join you—right away or down the road.

In other words, I want you to lead by example. That may require you to do some of your own cooking. If your mom is kind enough to prepare healthier food for you, she will obviously save time by cooking larger amounts of this food for the entire family. I've witnessed some great stories, in which once the son began to eat more healthfully, everyone else in the family did, too. It's not a mystery: The more people there are surrounding you who eat wisely, the more likely you are to stay true to your diet. The same goes for your buddies—training hard *and* eating well together will help you be more consistent with the Get Strong! plan.

At the same time, prepare yourself to have to do it all on your own. Prepare for your family and friends to call you a health freak, but instead of allowing them to tempt you left and right with junk, remain disciplined. I guarantee you that once they begin to see the fast changes that you make—leaner muscle, less body fat, more energy in your day and your exercise—with this new way of eating, the teasing comments will turn into questions like, "How'd you do that?"

THE TOP TWELVE KEYS TO GOOD EATING AND GREAT MUSCLE!

Training puts you on your way to developing the muscular physique you've been dreaming about. Eating right helps you get all the way there. Your V-12 engine needs premium fuel if you want to start and finish every workout strong, plus get to everything else you hope to accomplish that day. Here are the keys to eating like a winner:

1. The One-Day Challenge: before you discover the ways to eat smart, commit right now to try it out for one day. Make it all the way through without eating any junk food, and you'll see it wasn't so hard. Take this challenge for a few days, and soon it will become a way of life.

2. Consume the Right Calories: steer clear of the big- and empty-calorie items like soda, candy, chips, fatty meats, oil-laden sauces, and so on, unless you want to become boat-sized. Instead, eat healthy varieties of everything and go easy on the dessert. Sugar, in general, means calories, so keep that in mind when you eat a low-fat dessert that may carry as many cals as (sometimes even more than) the regular dessert. In other words, it doesn't give you license to double up! If you want to drop some pounds, cut out the desserts and go low-fat six days a week.

3. Super Substitutions: rather than giving up certain foods you like, simply make some healthier substitutions, such as: skim milk for 2-percent, egg white omelet for regular omelet, chicken breast for chicken leg, top-round steak for T-bone, turkey burger for hamburger, tuna packed in water for tuna in oil, and whole-grain bread for white. In addition, low-fat versions exist for almost any food, from deli meats, cheeses, soups, and chips to ice cream and cookies.

4. Nuke or Nonstick It: to prepare food quickly without adding fat or losing the nutrients, use the microwave. Meanwhile, encourage your parents to get nonstick cookware so they don't need to add extra oil or butter to cook the food.

5. Five a Day: eat five servings a day of fruits and vegetables. The nutrients will prevent you from getting colds, plus they'll boost your energy. Keep them around instead of sugary snacks that send you into an energy crash a half hour later.

6. Breakfast: eat it, *always*. Skipping breakfast lowers your metabolism, or your ability to burn fat. Having a healthy one with whole-grain cereal or oatmeal, egg whites, whole-wheat toast, and fruits starts your day on the right foot, plus it provides you with enough energy to last until lunchtime.

7. The Dairy Alternative: an allergy to dairy is very common. If you have stomach cramping or bloating, or you produce mucus after consuming a dairy product, you're allergic. Fortunately, there are many great alternatives now, with soy or rice versions of milk, cheese, and ice cream. Try them out!

8. The Day Off: your muscles need a day to laze out, and your taste buds deserve a little decadence once in a while, too. I allow myself one day a week to eat whatever I want (as long as I don't go nuts), then I'm much less likely to cheat for the rest of the week. Pick your day!

9. Food Isn't Always the Answer: Being bored silly or feeling blue can send you right to the fridge, but to get away from thinking, "I need ice cream, I need ice cream," call a friend, read a book, or go outside to exercise. You may well discover that you really weren't hungry after all.

10. Stop Scarfing: if you're like me, you have a tendency to inhale your food when you're hungry. The problem with eating so fast is that your stomach becomes full

before your brain registers that it's full, and consequently you've overeaten. Like my wife, Tracey, still reminds me, slow it down! Chew your food well, enjoy the taste, and take sips of water. This will be easier to practice if you eat *before* you're so hungry that roadkill even looks appetizing.

11. Water's the Way: it's our most abundant resource and makes up almost 70 percent of our body mass, yet few of us drink enough water. Consume a minimum of eight to ten 8-ounce glasses a day—more on your training days.

12. Your Go-To Foods: when you're in doubt about what to have at any meal, at any time, go for lean protein with some vegetables. If these staples are part of most of your meals, you can't go wrong.

▪ Three Body Types, Three Different Ways of Eating ▪

Are you built like a marathoner, an offensive lineman, or a wrestler? Thanks to our genetics, we fall into one of these three body types—also called ectomorphs, endomorphs, and mesomorphs. Ectomorphs tend to be lean and lanky. Because they rapidly burn up anything they eat, building muscle takes more work than it does for the other guys. However, they're often swift and have impressive endurance levels. Endomorphs, on the other hand, put on weight and muscle more easily. As a result, they're often very strong. Achieving muscle definition and a low body-fat percentage, though, prove more challenging. Mesomorphs are usually muscular and strong, and their bodies respond quickly to training. Because of such rapid gains, however, they can push themselves too hard, too fast.

As you see, regardless of which body type you have, some physical gains occur more easily, while others require more effort to develop—each type has its own challenges. When I was fourteen years old, I had no idea what an endomorph was, let alone the fact that I was one. I was aware of my chubby body, though, and I figured that was just the way I was meant to be. The fact that I considered a PB&J, chips, and a soda to be a tiny snack probably didn't help! Training hard and eating smart changed it all. Suddenly, instead of giving in to my body's tendency to gain fat, I took advantage of my ability to gain muscle—to the point where that tendency was no longer even visible!

I urge you to harness your own physique's abilities until they override the undesired tendencies. To maximize that ability, follow my Get Strong! workout four days a week, then eat according to your body type. In general, aim for one gram of protein per pound of body weight. Unlike carbs or fats, only protein contains the nitrogen and amino acids necessary for building muscle tissue.

Carbs, meanwhile, supply you with energy. In fact, it's what your muscles run on, whether you're going for a long bike ride or doing heavy bench presses. Therefore, 60 to 70 percent of your food intake should be carbs. The best variety are complex carbohydrates—like pasta, rice, potatoes, and whole grains—which have more healthy nutrients. Ectos and mesos can basically get away with eating as many as they want, but the endo should stick with the low-glycemic index (see below) variety. The endo should also do more cardio than the others if he wants to trim down.

TO LOSE FAT, EAT LIKE G.I. JACK

Joe wants to lose fat and drop weight, so he stops eating carbohydrates like bread, pasta, and potatoes, while jacking up his protein intake. Sure enough, within weeks, he's shrunk. But there's a big problem with this approach: It saps him of his physical and mental energy as a result of the low carbs, while his kidneys are overtaxed by the high amounts of protein. Plus, the only reason Joe's lost the weight in the first place is because he's eating fewer calories—a strategy that you can use with both carbs and protein, but one that will wear you out quickly.

Jack has a much better idea, since he knows it's really the *kind* of carbs you eat—and not the quantity—that makes the real difference with weight gain. In fact, he loses just as much weight, yet he doesn't restrict his calories and actually experiences a boost in energy rather than a drop. How? He knows about the glycemic index (or G.I.). Simply put, the G.I. measures how fast your body processes a carbohydrate food and gives it a ranking from 1 to 100. Foods that break down quickly after you eat them—thereby making you hungry again sooner—get a high G.I. number, while carbs that take longer to digest earn a lower G.I.

So, if you choose foods low on the G.I. scale, your belly will get full more quickly and stay full much longer—which means you won't be tempted to stuff your face every time you sit down to eat! A study in the medical journal *Pediatrics* gives you the overwhelming evidence: overweight teenage guys ate a whopping 81 percent more after a high-glycemic meal than after one with a low-glycemic index.

The trick, then, is finding which foods rank low versus high. Because it's confusing to figure out which foods belong in which camp, go to www.glycemicindex.com or www.mendosa.com/gilists.htm for more information. Keep in mind that refined, starch-laden carbs like corn chips, French fries, and cookies are on the high end—which explains why you can't have just one! You can always add protein, a little bit of fat, and fiber to bring the G.I. down as well.

Here's a small list of the better G.I. options for different food types:

Swap This High-G.I. Food for . . .	This Better Low-G.I. Food
French baguette, 95	mixed-grain bread, 48
Rice Chex, 89	oatmeal, 49
instant rice, 90	boiled white rice, 58
raisins, 64	apple, 38
rice noodles, 92	fettuccine (not overcooked), 32
baked potato, 85	sweet potato, 54
pretzels, 81	popcorn, 55

Understanding the G.I. can also help you a lot athletically. A couple of hours before your event or workout, take in low-G.I. foods that give you prolonged energy. Less than an hour afterward, meanwhile, is the best (and only!) time to eat those high on the scale to reload your carbohydrate stores in your muscles, which aids your recovery.

▪ Teenage Wasteland ▪

You hear the old Who song from my generation, and you think of drugged-out losers. Well, here I'm referring to drugged-*up* losers—the ones abusing steroids and other "performance-enhancing" drugs (such as growth hormone and insulin). In the mad search for more muscle and athletic power, many guys' are guilty of using a lot more than good nutrition. Performance-enhancing drug abuse is widespread in bodybuilding and in many other sports. But it's a very dangerous and destructive route, not only because it constitutes cheating and is banned by every major sport (except for bodybuilding, which tells you something!), but also because it wrecks your goals and your body.

I witnessed this firsthand in L.A. at age nineteen. For years I ate, drank, and slept the "Mr. America" dream. Through sheer determination and hard work, in my training and in my diet, I had transformed myself from a chubby kid into 245 pounds of manmade rock—or at least so I thought! Naively, I thought that was how everybody did it. So you can imagine my disappointment when I walked into the first serious bodybuilding gym in L.A. There, I saw guys I'd be competing against in the Mr. Teenage Los Angeles contest. These guys *my age* had tree trunk–sized muscles and worked out all day without seeming to tire. How was I going to catch up? I was already doing all I could.

One competitor gave me a scary answer: "Jake, you'll never make it without steroids," he said. Huh? I'd barely heard of them where I was from. I didn't want to believe it, but as I ran across the more competitive bodybuilders, it became an obvious truth. However, there was no way on Earth I'd take drugs. I believed in building muscles the natural way and keeping my body pure. Plus, you could forget the needle in the buttissimo!

A WORD ON SUPPLEMENTS

You're probably curious about the supplements hyped in the muscle magazines. Many are just that: hype. A few others, however, are worth considering, just as long as they're not used as a substitute for a well-balanced diet.

In the worthwhile column are a multimineral and protein powder. A multimineral is helpful if you didn't get your five servings of fruits and/or veggies that day. Protein powder is convenient to have on hand to throw into a fruit shake, if it looks like you're not going to have too much other protein that day.

On the other side of the fence sit the many others that will either give you nothing, or give you trouble. They include any product categorized as a thermogenic (which contains unnaturally high levels of stimulants, such as ephedra or Ma Huang), a prohormone (which contains steroid-like androgens), or a diurectic (which can cause unhealthy levels of dehydration). In addition, any product that attempts to mimic insulin or growth hormone (two very popular bodybuilding drugs that are very dangerous) is equally bad news for your body.

Deciding not to get on steroids meant I wouldn't be able to compete in bodybuilding, but that didn't stop me from trying. I'd worked so hard for so long, I was at least going to enter a couple of contests. In order to drop weight and get ripped for each competition, I cut out carbs—which meant I had zero energy and drooled a lot. Standing on stage next to these behemoths at the Mr.

Teenage Los Angeles contest I thought I'd get blown offstage by the air-conditioning fans! I finished fifth; the guy who won was on "the juice."

Next, at the Mr. Southern California contest, I had regained some of my lost muscle while remaining pretty well defined. This time, with my Go-To Grams in the crowd, I finished second. Again, the guy who won was a 'roider. It was a tough blow to take, but I realized that if taking steroids was the only way to win these bodybuilding contests, then I was in the wrong line of work. Just like that, I waved good-bye to my Mr. America dreams. Suddenly, it was no longer an ultimate goal that fit me anymore. In its place came far greater things—things that I couldn't have imagined if I hadn't decided not to take steroids.

According to my friend Dr. Bob Goldman, writer of *Death in the Locker Room—Steroids and Sports* and *The "E" Factor*, it looks much the same today. Oral anabolic steroids are the most common form of performance drugs, while some use the old method of injecting the drugs. Growth hormone and insulin aren't as widespread because of the higher cost. Overall, as many as 8 percent of high school athletes use a performance drug of some kind.

I urge you to never be one of them. Perhaps you envy the monsters in the muscle magazines, but you should know that these guys have paid the ultimate price for their bloated physiques: They've compromised their health. Not only do you court disaster—for instance, steroids can inhibit growth in young athletes, cause sterility and impotence, make you bald, increase your heart attack risk, create kidney tumors, and so on—but you cheat your sport and, most of all, yourself. You will feel so much better knowing you did it the old-fashioned way, with food, rather than by resorting to drugs that might make you look more muscular on the outside but will certainly ruin your insides.

By following my guidelines, you will gain muscle and/or become a great athlete through natural means, and the support for your success will emerge from the all-positive sources of good food and Go-To People. Nothing takes the place of hard work, nor is anything as rewarding as knowing you did it the right way. Once you're able to bench press 235 pounds by yourself, think of all the other things you can accomplish—from pancaking a defender on the field to acing your Spanish test and getting into your dream college. I can't wait for you to find out how much further you are going to go in sport and in life!

TAKE IT OUTSIDE

I'm not urging you—with your newfound strength and confidence—to physically challenge any rival who looks at you cross-eyed. You're smarter than that, and in the outside world that you're about to enter, it's more about flexing your brain than your biceps. Fortunately, you have soaked up the lessons in this book, and have felt and seen for yourself the powerful connection between getting stronger physically *and* mentally. Some work remains, however, if you want to prosper beyond your high school days.

Right now, you probably live in a small community—even if it's part of a big city—that revolves around school, relatives, and friends. When you finish high school, all of that changes in a flash. Suddenly, you're thrust into the world—going to college, gaining independence from your parents, landing a job, making money, finding the perfect woman for you, and marrying her!

Those prospects will either excite you or scare the heck out of you. (Especially that last one!) You will be ready for every step, however, because you're going to take everything in your life to the next level—your belief in yourself, your strength, your leadership, your goals, and your support system. To make that happen and to tap your ever-growing potential, there are some things left to work on before you close this chapter of your life (and this book)! They include solidifying a good reputation, expanding yourself to study new ideas and team up with new people, picking up the pace with your tasks and goals, and creating your own momentum.

Mastering these abilities and skills in your current environment will serve you very well, for not only will you experience greater successes in the immediate future, but the big future down the road will be much less daunting. Consequently, unlike the countless others who enter the post–high school existence blindfolded and unprepared, you will know what to expect and how to conquer every challenge. After all, you haven't invested all your time and energy into making yourself a strong leader, just to stumble into the unknown. You're going to be ready!

▪ Rep It Up ▪

One's reputation tends to stick, as that girl who is rumored to have slept around in ninth grade knows all too well! So take it seriously when it comes to yours. Before you walk through any door—from the one belonging to the college admission lady to the parents of your potential girlfriend—chances are that your reputation was there first. Your past actions, especially the praiseworthy (you wrote a great application essay) and the boneheaded (this girl's father knows you from your days as the neighborhood mailbox vandal), are now paying off big time or punishing you plenty.

Consider your future actions carefully, and either keep building or rebuild that rep. How do you do that? It starts with people: Leave a good impression on every person with whom you come into contact from now on. If there is bad blood with somebody, clear it up before it leaves a stain on your reputation.

Even if you have a seriously bad reputation, it's never too late. We live in a very forgiving country, where the past is easily forgotten so long as the present offers a new and improved you. From the president of the United States to sport stars to members of your own family, there are many examples of a person who has committed bad acts only to bounce back stronger and more respected, because he or she was courageous enough to face these problems square on. Perhaps you are known as a troublemaker, but if you have the guts first to deal with the source of these acts, then apologize to those you have hurt or offended and tell them you're a changed man—they will want to believe you. Then it's up to you to prove it!

Continue to be a leader wherever you go. For instance, when someone needs help, be the first person to offer assistance. Leadership exists as strongly in these situations as anywhere else. Perhaps you like to be described as "clever" or "hardworking," but "trustworthy" and "good" tell more about what other people really think about you.

POWER HABIT: *Build Values That Will Never Let You, or Others, Down*

Make a conscious effort to develop values that will always keep you centered and in control; they are your anchors. Some of the values that will serve you well include having integrity, when you become the guy you want people to think you are; being optimistic, when being a positive force is not just for yourself, but for everyone around you; and achieving balance, when nothing will throw you off your stride because you have a strong mix of challenging goals and close relationships.

You may inherit these values from your parents or from others around you, or you may choose to work on your very own. Here's a great way to come up with the perfect "value system" for you:

1. Make a list: write down the values that you believe are most important to you in the present and future. Examples include academic success, love, athletic domination, laughter, recognition, wealth.

2. Rank them: place each of the values you wrote down in their order of importance.

3. Describe what is required: write a paragraph for each value explaining what it will take for you to attain these values.

4. Give yourself the once-over: have you made it hard or easy to develop these values? Do you have to ace every class and letter in three varsity sports in order to have the academic and athletic success you want? Are you more focused on doing well in one or just a few subjects like history and English? Is getting an athletic scholarship for one sport the most important to you? Don't set the bar too high at first; instead, give yourself a realistic shot at attaining a semblance of each value soon, then plan on developing each more and more. Remember: For some of these values, such as love, there's always more where *that* came from!

To gain the respect and admiration of others, carry yourself with an air of quiet confidence and let your values shine. People can't help but be impressed by such an aura of calm, competence, and essential goodness. Why is this important? Because the way in which you are viewed plays a major role in determining your future—from getting admitted to the right college, chosen by the right girl, or hired for the right job.

For example, if you prize academic success, you need to act the part: sit at the front of the class, communicate often with your teacher, anticipate what each class period and each test will be about, form a study group with a couple of classmates, and do your homework—plus a little extra. Practicing all those steps also puts you on the fast track to making that value a big part of you. To cement your athletic reputation, similar steps are needed: training with weights, doing sport-specific drills, having good nutritional habits, practicing hard, and becoming a leader whom your coach and team can always rely on. Doing these things will add to your athletic value, and others—from your teammates to college scouts—will take notice and have confidence in your abilities.

Your parents, teachers, and friends, and especially the Go-To People among them, may have great expectations for you. However, their expectations should never be as high as your own. If you are a perfectionist in all that you attempt, then you can never stop halfway in your pursuit of a goal or value. At the same time, don't take yourself too seriously. Have a sense of humor about yourself, so you can poke fun at yourself rather than letting other guys do it for you! Work on your shortcomings, but laugh at them as well.

One shortcoming that is never acceptable, though, is looking like a slob. If you look like you don't care about yourself, then why should anyone else care about you? I'm not recommending primping yourself into *GQ* man, but being clean-shaven and wearing clean clothes are a good start! You're feeling good on the inside and getting your body into great shape, so why not match that with how you present yourself? Just like you create your own group of friends to hang out with, create your own style as well. Put all this together, and everyone from pretty girls to future employers will be knocking at your door.

Creating a good reputation has been a focus of mine since I was fourteen, when I realized I no longer wanted to be known as chubby, stuttering Jake. Now my reputation is my business. There's no way I'd be able to make as many deals as I do if my business partners viewed me as untrustworthy, unlucky, or incompetent, for example. My fitness and motivational products, including this book, won't sell as well if I become out-of-shape or stuck in a scandal! Don't worry, I will never allow those kinds of things to happen!

▪ Reach Out to Reap Rewards ▪

As your abilities and confidence grow, so does your ability to face challenges all by yourself. While that may seem admirable and leaderlike, you will end up going down a much longer road than necessary. Instead, to be a solid leader, realize that your intended success doesn't only involve you, but also all those who team up with you! With that team, learn how to delegate authority and share your challenge. Suddenly, the most difficult challenges will seem easy.

Let's say you want to make a small film. Your family, friends, teachers, and fellow students provide you with a huge recruiting base for this project. When they see that you're working on a dream, they're apt to want to lend a hand. If you're struggling to keep your dream alive—raising money, finding locations, getting actors—they will admire that. Moreover, perhaps they can see what's in it for them and be almost as excited as you are—helped along by your showing them exactly what is in it for them! Also, you can help them with their projects so that what you accomplish together will be even greater.

POWER HABIT: *Play Ball!*

These are your best years to play sports and enjoy it—being part of a team week after week, building great friendships, playing in front of crowds, having adults ask you how the next game will go. The individual athletic accomplishments are great, but the bond that you create with your teammates—through practicing hard, going on the road, eating meals together, and winning or losing—is what makes the experience one that is not to be missed.

Playing on a team will teach you how to *work* together to achieve a single aim; becoming a leader on that team teaches you how to help the many personalities *stay* together and continually improve, in play and in friendship. In fact, it's where many prominent people today, from CEOs to politicians, first began their training. If an organized sport isn't your thing, you can still have the same experience with a group of friends who frequently do an activity together, such as skateboarding or playing in a band.

Throughout it all, your most vital teammate is your Go-To Person(s). When you don't have anywhere else to turn, your Go-To will be there, willing and able to help. They want you to put your potential to great use because they, too, want to see you achieve your dreams. Whenever you seem to hit a ceiling and can't seem to go any further, he or she will find a way to elevate you. After high school, the role of your future Go-To People becomes even more important and can make the difference in your career.

Before you start thinking of what specific job you want later in life, however, ask yourself what general interests you have now; then determine your field of interest. To boost your chances of success in this field, get in touch with all its inner workings, from the people making things happen to news in the field, to technical information. If you really want to navigate successfully, then start studying up on the territory now; that includes walking through any door that opens—after all, you can always walk back out. Jump on any opportunity that shows itself, because you never know what will take you to the next level.

Let's say human rights are your passion, so you begin to read all the human rights journals, pay close attention to our government's policies, observe the international groups, and find out which colleges have an international relations program. Maybe you run across an offer to join a respected human rights organization as an intern, and you take it! The more you know about your potential field, the further you will progress within it.

▪ Step Up the Pace ▪

Imagine this: You set out on a thirty-minute run from your front porch, going at a steady pace around your neighborhood, yet are disappointed when you finish back at home. Why? You haven't sweated enough, burned enough calories, made enough use of your energy stores—you name it. Not because you stopped at thirty minutes, as that's plenty of time for a great cardiovascular workout. Rather, because you never picked up the pace. The same can be true for the rest of your day and beyond. You're tasting success and rolling along nicely, but don't you want more? I know you do.

One method to accelerate your rate of success is keeping several balls in the air. Sometimes, through no fault of your own, a project or goal of yours won't pan out—and the ball drops. However, if you have other projects and goals that you're also working on, you'll barely skip a beat. Use your overload of energy by dispersing it across an array of projects and tasks.

Without knowing it, you probably already engage in this juggling act in your daily life—you take a full load of classes, play different sports, attend different after-school meetings, talk with your teachers and coaches, spend time with your friends and family, have a part-time job, and date a couple of girls. In addition to all these things are your goals, so instead of tossing up a few balls, you're juggling dozens! That overload of energy has dwindled to nothing, and your day closes before you've accomplished the things you had on your mind when it started.

You can change that by prioritizing each ball. As a result, your less important balls may drop to the ground, but your eyes remain locked on the essential ones. In much the same way, the juggler who tosses up a few breakable possessions along with some regular objects is going to do his best not to let the breakable ones smash on the ground.

The same should be true of you. Evaluate which classes, sports, people, and future prospects are the most important, and place these at the top of your list. Save the others for when you have the time and energy to deal with them well. Stay focused on what you want—your goal of becoming a writer, doing well in your history and English classes, spending time with your family and group of friends, getting ready for your upcoming basketball season, and asking out the cute girl in the class below you. Even if you fumble a couple of these "balls," you'll be ahead of the game.

POWER HABIT: *More Speed, More Success*

Another route to your goals is the direct, fast one. Speed, after all, has a lot to do with success—and not just in sports. Soon you'll realize that life is lived on the autobahn, where the guys who get more things done in a shorter amount of time are the ones who rule the highway. Here are the ways to gain the speed you need:

1. When opportunity knocks, act fast: windows of opportunity often close quickly. You catch a beautiful girl's eye at the movie theater, then see her again in the lobby afterward? Go up and introduce yourself. Otherwise, it might be the last time you see that pretty face! Have an opportunity to get an internship in the field you want to join one day? Take it!

2. Be a day early and never a minute late: when anything is expected of you, surprise them by showing up or getting it done early. If it's a class or your date, get there before your expected arrival time. If it's your homework, finish it way before it's due. I'm not recommending a slapdash effort, however; make sure that if you get it done early, that it's because you also started early. When it comes to your own deadlines, meet them. Training at 5 P.M.? Don't be late. Finish that book by Sunday night? Get to reading!

3. Underpromise and overdeliver: you believe in yourself and in your capacity for tremendous feats, but don't broadcast that whatever needs to be done will be ready in no time and, what's more, in great shape! Instead, give them a realistic date when it will be done, then push yourself to finish it *sooner.* Also, if someone expects you to do a good job, do a *great* job!

4. Never give yourself time to second-guess yourself: you made the decision, now stick with it. Don't stand there scratching your head and saying, "Maybe I should have . . ." You decided to write your essay on the politics of music; you decided to take Suzanne to the prom; you decided to accept the scholarship to the University of Texas. The decision was made for a good reason, so follow it up with effort immediately. If it turns out that it was a bad one, at least you saw it through. Usually, though, your relentless work will turn even the most shaky decisions into solid ones.

In general, the benefit to picking up the pace is that it increases the likelihood of your achieving your goals. Sometimes roadblocks will slow you down, or your goal doesn't work for you in the end. In any case, you will have flown right by the distractions and doubts, so you'll know if it is right for you.

Don't forget: The last stretch in your pursuit of success is the most critical. Anyone who plays a sport can tell you the last few minutes of the game are the ones that matter most. The same holds true with everything else. Finish strong: the workout, the essay, the work shift, the date! Leave it on a good note; leave it on a strong note.

▪ Go with Your Flow ▪

Rather than going with the flow, you must create your own flow. I want you to be so energized by your goals that you completely forget about everything else around you, especially the potential obstacles and distractions. That allows you to reach the rare state where your talents and abilities are used at the highest levels, and one good thing happens after the next.

To get the flow going, stop being a person who *waits* for something to happen; instead, be someone who *makes* things happen. Few great things in life come to you without real effort. If you used to lie in bed, dreaming of having big muscles, then next you should start training to make those muscles. Soon training will get in your blood, and you'll feel it positively affect everything in your life!

My flow began in my basement, pumping weights. First, it began to affect the way I felt about myself, the way I looked, the way I ate. Then, it improved my dealings with the outside world, from friends and girls to teachers and coaches. That's why every morning I lift weights first thing, because it gets me right back into the flow. Physically, the blood is circulating and the adrenaline is kicking in; mentally, I think about my goals for the day. In my business, whenever I put a major deal together, I begin turning on the flow by determining whom I can call and what I can do to make the deal work.

When you attend a music concert or play, you will notice whether or not the entertainers are in a flow. The musician may be on such a roll that he plays inspired stuff for three straight hours with hardly a break, or the actors are clicking so well on stage that you forget that this isn't real. Meanwhile, in sports, it's common to see some athletes so "on" that it seems they can do no wrong.

Perhaps your flow will also start with training, or it could be some altogether different goal, such as wanting to be a marine biologist or computer engineer. Whatever it is, your goal can fill you with such intensity and excitement that you sense those emotions carrying over to other parts of your life. Anytime you were working on a task when you suddenly realized that you had no idea where the time had gone or that your mom had been calling your name for five minutes, you were in a flow.

For that flow to really get moving, it must have somewhere to go. This means that you need to have a plan in place that connects all the goals and important things in your life—including your family, friends, studies, sports, and future prospects. If any one of these things is out of order, the flow might come to an abrupt halt. Bringing your goals, talents, and interests into all sectors of your life, however, will often prevent that lapse from occurring. For example, perhaps science isn't your bag and whenever you do your science homework, your flow instantly stops—but if your goal is to get good grades, you will learn to enjoy the work.

When you truly feel satisfied with an achievement, you can't wait to keep performing new and different feats. You've experienced the "flow feeling," and anything seems possible. Once in a while, though, you won't do as well, and that feeling will seem to vanish, along with your confidence. Please be aware that moments like these are normal. Fortunately, you know what to do to get it going again: namely, keep listening to your interests and don't stop using your talents in the big chase of your ultimate goal.

You'll be amazed by how much you're capable of when in a flow. In the workout, you suddenly lift more weight and feel like you can go forever. Or treat a high-pressure day that includes a family fight, a tough math test, and a big game as a unique opportunity rather than as a day to be forgotten, and you'll not only survive it but experience success in every situation. Sure enough, you will resolve the fight between you and your sister, know all the answers on the test, and score the winning points for your team!

REALITY CHECK: *Get Ready for Your Call*

You will find that being prepared instantly raises your level of success in all your pursuits, both today and in the future. Your English teacher, who gives a pop essay on the book you just read, will give you a passing grade if you skimmed the book—but if you pored over it and thought carefully about the themes and characters, you will write something worthy of an A. At your track team's big meet, you will do okay if you've at least done the minimum that your coach has asked of you—but if instead you used almost every minute of practice time over the past months to improve your track skills, you will dominate out there!

The lesson is simple: Always be prepared, mentally and physically, for any challenge. Why? Because you never know when that challenge is going to arrive. Anyone in the Army Reserves has to be prepared to serve our country whenever the government decides it's necessary. Reservists are required to be ready mentally to endure war and physically to carry out their duties. Their chances of survival and success are much better if they remain in a state of readiness for such an undertaking. You, too, must be poised for any struggle that you may face, in school, on the field, when running for class president, or in any other competitive endeavor.

As you know, life is not played on the sidelines. Therefore, you must be ready to be put into the game at any moment. Daunting challenges don't come along every day, but neither do great opportunities! You must not only accept them, but prosper with each one. Look at my buddy Harrison Ford: He met some serious challenges in the early days by becoming a carpenter to support his family, all the while studying the craft he really loved—acting. One day while hammering in floorboards at MGM Studios, his big opportunity for stardom arrived—the role of a lifetime in *Star Wars*. He pounced on it!

I want *you* to pounce on all your challenges and opportunities. If you keep working toward your goals, developing your skills and your individuality, then there will be many of them—and many people who will offer them because they can see for themselves that you're ready. You've heard the expression "prepare for greatness"; now do just that. It will be on its way!

▪ The Don't Quit! Journey ▪

As you have already begun to learn, the great thing about having goals is not achieving them—it's the journey you take to get there. Life becomes an adventure when you are aiming for small goals every day and big goals down the road. Consider the most successful sport experience you've been a part of, whether it ended in a championship or you and your team simply improved by the season's end. While the end result was great, the best part was getting there—the practices, great plays, playing game after game, bonding with your teammates—toward that celebratory end.

My big goal as a teenager was to become Mr. America. Just the thought of claiming that prize fueled me for years, as I spent countless hours building up my body into that of the muscular guy who I thought deserved that prize. By the time I got close to that goal, though, I realized that much bigger and better things were in store for me.

My Mr. America dream took me on a great trip that I will never forget. It was all unforgettable—all the hard work and dedication it required, the lessons I learned about training and eating, the positive responses I got from people around me, and the fact that it persuaded me to move to L.A., where I still live today. Most of all, it helped transform me from a fat, stuttering kid into a confident, fit young man. Yep, I owe that dream plenty.

You, too, have dreams that will transform you way before you reach them. Turn them into distinct goals, and they put you in the driver's seat to controlling your own destiny. Every morning, feel good looking in that mirror and start your day off by saying, "I can." Then believe that you can do whatever you hope to accomplish.

Ultimately, the single most important reason for your success—beyond facing your fears, seeing failure as a stepping stone to success, becoming a leader—is commitment. Be committed, and go where and do what you want. Stay committed, and you never run out of energy in your relentless pursuit of your goals. One of my mottoes is "Go Big or Stay Home," which means, commit to it or don't bother—show that commitment in your training, at school, and for your future!

Your life is not about success and failure, praise and criticism. It's about being in charge and looking ahead to a positive future, no matter what happens to you—including the worst defeat or harshest criticism. You will become the sort of person you have always wanted to be, for whom success and praise come naturally.

I urge you to work hard and *enjoy* the task at hand—gaining muscle, getting a top G.P.A., landing a great summer job, dating the perfect girl for you. Achieving these goals will be extremely worthwhile and will set you up for even bigger challenges. Many guys reach a level of success and happiness and then just stay there; you will keep moving up. Just as the methods required to meet those current challenges never stay the same, neither do you. You might want a leaner, quicker body instead of a bulky one; you might prefer a summer job at the United Nations; you might decide to apply to that Ivy League college that nobody thinks you'll get into. Achieving "staying power" means you never stop progressing!

I've spent time with some of the most famous people in the world, people whom I had watched on the big screen as a teenager. Let me tell you something that I want you to remember: They're no different from you or me. Decide, like I did then, that you are going to do what you love and that you will make it work. You're not going to take "no" for an answer. What are you waiting for? Slap this book shut and go to it! Don't Quit! Ever!

INDEX

INDEX

154

Jake Steinfeld is best known as the man behind "Body by Jake." He created the industry of Personal Fitness Training and built Body by Jake into a household icon, symbolic of strength, motivation, and ideal physical stature. Jake created the world's first 24-hour fitness television network and also starred in his own sitcom, *Big Brother Jake*. He is the founder of the nonprofit Don't Quit! Foundation and of Major League Lacrosse.

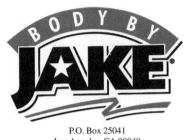

P.O. Box 25041
Los Angeles, CA 90049

**For more information on
Body by Jake Weight Training Equipment,
Nutritional Supplements, Fitness Videos and Motivation,
please visit us at www.bodybyjake.com**